IF
CANCER
is a
GIFT

Can I

RETURN

It?

From Grief to Healing

AGALIA BAKER MSN, FNP-BC-Ret

If Cancer is a Gift, Can I Return it?
From Grief to Healing

Edited by Laurie Knight
Cover Design by: Kristina Edstrom

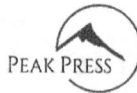

PEAK PRESS

An Imprint for GracePoint Publishing (www.GracePointPublishing.com)
GracePoint Matrix, LLC
624 S. Cascade Ave, Suite 201, Colorado Springs, CO 80903
www.GracePointMatrix.com   Email: Admin@GracePointMatrix.com
SAN # 991-6032

A Library of Congress Control Number has been requested and is pending.

ISBN: (Paperback): 978-1-961347-22-9
eISBN: 978-1-961347-23-6

Books may be purchased for educational, business, or sales promotional use.
For bulk order requests and price schedule contact:
Orders@GracePointPublishing.com

Table of Contents

A Letter to Agalia from Dr. Makhoul

Steven Covey once said, "To touch the soul of another human being is to walk on holy ground." Reading your book is walking on holy ground. Your account of your cancer roller-coaster is unique in the sense that you have been there and lived every minute of it, which gives you credibility beyond any doubt. You opened your heart and allowed the readers into the most intimate details of your personal history, your fears, hopes, weaknesses and strengths.

Sharing the lessons learned with current and future breast cancer patients responds to an unfulfilled need. This is a book about the "Knowhow" to become a cancer veteran. It should be a recommended reading to all breast cancer patients, or in fact any cancer patient, going through this experience. Health care profess-sionals and people living with or taking care of cancer patients will benefit immensely from your testimony.

You have weaved masterfully your breast cancer story with a reflective and analytical component of the different stages of grief. I am sure that writing about your lived experience was therapeutic. For the "unbelievers" of the suffering and pain that is the alpha-betical reality of the cancer journey, you took their fingers and put them right in the wound. You did your homework too. You searched for possible solutions to guide the cancer travelers through their journey without being forceful or too assertive about what might work for others.

You highlighted the uniqueness of every human being. I totally agree with you. Our "value" is intrinsic because we have been born into this world. We do not need any additional attributes to earn it. This is true in a spiritual and physical sense. No need to elaborate on the spiritual aspect here. Our physical uniqueness is manifested by the fact that everybody interacts with cancer treatments in a unique and different way. While the side effects of the treatments are numerous and not all will happen to everybody, the intensity of these side effects is variable from one patient to the other. As physicians sitting on the other side of the table, we try to provide our patients with a detailed explanation of the different treatment options with their potential benefits and potential side effects. And I learned a long time ago to include "no treatment" as an option. And we ask them to choose.

However, as you rightly mentioned, here is the problem. The patients are asked to make rational decisions at a time when their rational brain is shut down. Their eyes don't see, and their ears don't hear. Hence the importance of other sets to eyes and ears like family members, friends, and loved ones to be present. Nobody can—or should—go through the cancer journey alone. The personal support system should be called on early to make sure that it is in place when needed. The professional support system is a must, not a luxury. Professional counseling and cancer support groups should be a part of any cancer program.

Cancer is synonymous with loss in all its dimensions. Other than the loss of body parts or functions, job, partners, or good time etc., it is a loss of control over our own bodies. Even when these losses are not major, the patient is left with this uncontrolled intrusive idea of the cancer coming back. This anxiety manifests itself as post-traumatic stress disorder and may poison the patients' lives for years. Your discussion of this aspect of the

If Cancer is a Gift, Can I Return It?

cancer journey is deep and relevant to many cancer patients. Your proposed solutions will resonate with most of our patients.

Even though we can't control what life throws at us, we still can control our response to it. Your attitude in this matter resonates with the main conclusion that Viktor Frankl, an Auschwitz survivor, had reached after being in concentration camps for three years. In his famous book, *Man's Search for Meaning* he says, "Everything can be taken from a man but one thing: the last of the human freedoms—to choose one's attitude in any given set of circumstances, to choose one's own way." And about the meaning of life, "Ultimately, man should not ask what the meaning of his life is, but rather must recognize that it is he who is asked. In a word, each man is questioned by life; and he can only answer to life by answering for his own life; to life he can only respond by being responsible." I would say, response-able. And he concludes, "So live as if you were living already for the second time and as if you had acted the first time as wrongly as you are about to act now!"

I think you have a vivid imagination and fantastic sense of humor that captures the essence of the moment and helps you and others diffuse the tension inherent to difficult situations in the cancer context. I still have the "Bionic Boob" comic that you have conceived following our discussion. It draws laughter and sense of empathy from all those who see it in my office.

Your book is a Manifesto for Emotional Support. It is shedding bright light on the "invisible" gorilla in the room, which is patients' emotional journey with cancer. We can't claim any-more that nobody has talked about it. I heard it loud and clear, and my understanding of the issue deepened after I read it!

Dedication

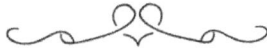

This book is dedicated to Dr. Issam Makhoul. He saw his patients for who they were, not their cancer. He never lost sight of their value. He gave me hope, encouragement, and was my greatest cheerleader for every micro-achievement. He showed me kindness when I needed it, and he challenged me to put to paper what I was feeling during my lowest times. Without him, this book would not have been possible. I totally "blame" him for this.

If Cancer Is a Gift, Can I Return It?

When I decided to write a book about the breast cancer experience, this title, *If Cancer Is a Gift, Can I Return It?* was the first thing that came to me. Every time I heard someone say my cancer was my gift or wake-up call, it hurt. I hadn't lived a perfect life, but I survived what was thrown at me the best I could. To think of cancer being my so-called gift is to believe I deserved pain, trauma, loss of my breasts, and everything else that came afterward. Surely, I didn't deserve this lump of coal at Christmastime.

When I was diagnosed with breast cancer, I was devastated. I never wanted to believe it could happen to me. I was used to being on the other side of the equation as a nurse, helping women along the prevention, education, and medical routes. Suddenly, I was both a health care provider and a very unprepared patient. I was overwhelmed and so emotional I did not know what was happening to me. Because of the two-month wait between my diagnosis and the first step in treatment, a mastectomy, I had too much time on my hands to think. Most of the time that thinking was around 2 a.m. because insomnia was my new normal. I tortured myself with the horrors of my own imagination. I needed help and didn't know where to find it.

At the time I was diagnosed, Facebook support groups weren't mainstream yet, so I felt very alone. I knew precious few people personally who had experienced breast cancer, and I desperately needed someone to tell me it was going to be okay. But no one could do that for me because with breast cancer, there are no guarantees. Searching fruitlessly for a breast cancer survival guide to explain the mental and emotional chaos I experienced, I had the first thought that maybe I should write the book I was looking for.

In theory, my experience should have been an easy one. I had early detection of a type of cancer that showed promising results to certain chemotherapy agents. I was to have a single mastectomy with reconstruction. End of story. But things didn't work out that way for me. Everything turned out to be delivered the hard way. I agonized over whether I was making the "right" decision at every turn. From picking a breast surgeon and whether to have my healthy breast removed initially, to ending up with a nightmare reconstruction and finally having to have the implants out.

In addition, I experienced a scare on my "good boob" later that led me to choosing to remove it too. Finally, I had to make the choice to remove the implants knowing I wasn't a good candidate for another reconstruction procedure with no guarantees the removal would bring any relief. In the process, I lost my job, career, and a huge chunk of my identity. I lost use of my arms and shoulders due to inflammation and lived too many years in pain from them. I had to buy clothes I didn't like to camouflage my chest in styles based solely on being able to get in and out of them without raising my arms. Insomnia was my constant companion because I couldn't find a pain-free position to fall asleep. Looking back, I can see my stumbling through the getting-over-breast-cancer process making mistakes was exactly what I needed to grow, learn, heal, and write.

Only in hindsight did I realize there is one common denominator for every person experiencing a breast cancer diagnosis: the trauma of loss. Everyone diagnosed with breast cancer suffers multiple losses. While grief is most commonly associated with death of a loved one, it's a process people go through with any type of loss. With daily life challenges, it is easy to overlook the impact grief and the grieving process has in our lives.

Very much like the well-known stages of grief, loss associated with breast cancer seems to also have steps along a path, but most who experience breast cancer haven't been told what to expect, how they might feel, all the wrong things people may say, or other things only someone who has been through it would know. I am here to help readers navigate this journey because I was that person.

Once I realized the emotional chaos I experienced when diagnosed was the grief over the loss of the life I once had before cancer, everything made sense. With that loss, my future was irrevocably changed. Not only did I lose the life I once knew, but I also lost the dream of living to a ripe old age without the threat of cancer following me the rest of the way.

Now I can see that if I had acknowledged my grief at the time, I could have recognized that what I was feeling matched up with each of the stages of grief. And that what was happening to me was natural—predictable even. I imagine I could have relaxed my white-knuckle grip on myself with this earlier awareness. I placed impossible expectations on myself not understanding how truly futile they were.

For me, cancer wasn't a gift or a wake-up call, so I refuse to give cancer the credit for my growth and healing. That credit goes to me. My cancer was nothing but a catalyst for my faith and growth. When life throws us any catalyst for change, we have the choice to grow bitter or better. I chose better; cancer didn't choose for me. My lump of coal under pressure became a diamond where it could have just as easily burned to ash. It happened *because* of me and who I am, not cancer.

When something disastrous like cancer happens in a person's life, it is natural, even healthy, to look for something positive or good to come out of the situation. Many people learn their priorities need to change, they learn the value of saying no, or their perspectives on life pivot. All the changes can be good, but they are a result of who you are at heart, not cancer. To say cancer is your gift is to give it power over your life. Being without personal power, in my opinion, feels like living at the mercy of fate. I tried that and it didn't work out so well for me.

Good things can and will come as a result of experiencing cancer. However, cancer means change, which isn't always easy to weather. For me, change is awesome but only if it's my idea and I'm in full control of it; otherwise, I'm not a fan. I didn't want to give up my career but found that retirement has its positive side. Giving up my breasts was traumatic, but I discovered a freedom where my identity is not so tightly bound up in my body image.

Changes bring loss, and some of my losses brought gains. Superficial relationships fell away making room for stronger ones. Areas in my life showed up letting me know I was carrying too big a load and informing me it was time to let others carry their own crap. To get through breast cancer is to make "frenemies" with change. Sometimes change is hell, but it doesn't stay that way. It gets better. When you have gone through the darkest of nights, the new dawn is pretty amazing.

I hope that anyone reading this while actively undergoing cancer treatment is feeling well and will be seeing better days ahead. If treatment is in the rearview mirror but has still left the proverbial semi-truck tire tracks across you, I hope that you will see yourself with more compassion for the way you got through such a horrible ordeal. I'm glad you made it.

For those who are experiencing breast cancer in someone you love, I hope you find clarity in the emotional chaos of cancer that you and they are experiencing. The partners and loved ones of those going through breast cancer experience the challenges of grief right along with them. It must be even harder, in a way, to watch events unfold out of your control. For all the readers who are treating, caring for, and helping breast cancer patients in any way, thank you for being who you are.

I'm hoping through stories like mine, the medical society and the general public see that receiving a breast cancer diagnosis is a traumatic event requiring attention and respect. Regardless of prognostics and treatment protocols, a cancer diagnosis is a trauma that takes its toll from day one. A person's mental and emotional status is as vitally important to a healthy outcome as the physical body. No one should have to fall apart before receiving the support and guidance they need. Support systems need to be in place for anyone who wants it regardless of their socioeconomic status and ability to pay. Now is the time for a more compassionate change.

My greatest hope is that you discover yourself to be the most tremendous gift of all. Cancer can destroy many things you trusted and believed to be true, but you are the reason cancer cannot destroy you.

No one gets through this life without trauma. We adapt, build walls, hide, or try to be something we are not. Cancer destroys that fragile façade giving you the opportunity and freedom to be your beautiful, authentic self. It's your choice. You are an irreplaceable thread in the tapestry of all that is, with or without cancer. Your gift to yourself and the world is to drop all the constraints of past trauma that told you it was not safe to be yourself and be who you are at heart. You deserve the credit, not cancer. It was just a life challenge that brought the gift *of you* to the forefront. It really has nothing to do with cancer.

Be free.

Blindsided

As a nurse practitioner in women's health, I was supposed to *screen* women for breast cancer and teach preventive measures, not get it myself. Nevertheless, on May 17, 2011, I heard the words, "I'm sorry, it's cancer," and my life fell apart. My routine mammogram had become an unfathomable nightmare.

I was fifty-four years old and had—just three years earlier—started my expanded career as a nurse practitioner. Breast cancer wasn't in my plan. Whenever I envisioned my mortality or even how my life was to evolve, cancer was never in it. It never even crossed my radar. I had no obvious risk factors, no family history, my cancer was not hormonally triggered, and I had no known genetic mutations. There was no reason to suspect I would ever face getting this diagnosis.

Sometimes I joked about how I wanted to go at eighty-five when my parachute didn't open, but figured I would die of old age like so many in my family. Although I never bought into the dream that life was not full of incredible challenges, breast cancer wasn't supposed to be one of them. And yet it was.

Breast cancers vary widely in types, treatment modalities, staging or size, and whether it has gone to lymph nodes or elsewhere in the body. Then there is the process of grading which refers to the level of aggressiveness and prognosis.

My tumor was unusual in that it was not the more common hormonally triggered type found in women over fifty. Rather, my tumor tested positive for a protein called *human epidermal growth factor receptor 2* (HER2). Ultimately, too much of this protein causes an overgrowth of cancer cells. HER2 tumors are more aggressive but respond well to targeted chemotherapy; however, my tumor was graded at a 3, which is the most aggressive, fast-growing category. Since my tumor was two centimeters and had not progressed to the lymph nodes, I was given a diagnosis of stage 1, grade 3, ER neg., PR neg., HER2 positive breast cancer. All things considered, my prognosis was favorable, but having *any* kind of cancer is not reassuring news.

Trouble with my left breast was nothing new. In my mid-thirties, I developed a benign fluid-filled cyst there. Although it wasn't a precursor for cancer, after finding the cyst, I had regular exams as a preventive measure. Because of the cyst, which would sometimes reoccur, I became used to being called back for an ultrasound after a routine mammogram then being sent for a procedure to aspirate the cyst. It was no big deal.

When I received the call that my last mammogram required an ultrasound as follow-up to check a certain area, I wasn't bothered in the least. In fact, it was a good excuse to take a day off and explore a few shops after the procedure. The thought that it might be more than another fluid-filled cyst never entered my mind. I went to my appointment filled with optimism and anticipation of a good day.

My first clue that something was off was the look of the radiologist's face. The concern in his eyes told me this lump wasn't fluid filled as before. I was given an appointment to see a breast surgeon for a biopsy in a couple of days.

My years as a critical care nurse had taught me to always wait to react. I should get all the facts and see for myself what I was dealing with first. So, I put all thoughts about possibilities of what it *might* be on hold until I met with the doctor and the biopsy was completed.

My initial visit with my breast surgeon was good in that I felt she was both compassionate and competent. She ordered a few X-rays and a special biopsy—the stereotactic biopsy—which was more intense and painful than I had anticipated. Basically, I was placed face down on a platform table with a hole to drop my breast into. Then, the platform was raised nearly to the ceiling and two cold plates of something clamped onto my dangling breast. I was warned it would squeeze hard, and they weren't joking. Then a needle was injected into the lump to obtain a sample of the tissue. It felt like I took a bullet to the breast. Thankfully, it didn't last long. They released me and I couldn't get out of there fast enough. That evening, I received a call from my breast surgeon and my life was forever changed.

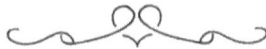

⁕

When I was fourteen, I loved to run. I ran tirelessly, my legs gliding over the distances as comfortably as if I were flying. There was such joy in seeing the blur of field grass beneath my feet as I ran. Then I got the worst sore throat of my life. Since I didn't see a doctor, I have no idea what caused the sore throat, nor did I receive any treatment. My lack of seeing a doctor was more about stressed parents, tough economic times, and a culture that promoted tough-it-out and tincture-of-time attitudes. In my home in the early '70s, doctors' visits were only considered if there were broken bones or a lot of blood. In fairness to my parents, I don't remember if I even told them about my sore throat.

Although I got better quickly, about three weeks later, my health plummeted. That's when I started running a low-grade fever at night that continued for a month. I became so weak I was unable to attend school and dropped to eighty-five pounds on my five-foot-three frame. It took me a year before I felt remotely normal, but I could never run again without exhaustion. Walking felt like I was wading through quicksand. Time passed, but I always felt like I was struggling to regain the joy of running, that joy of good health.

A career in nursing called me, and I answered the call when I entered the first nursing class of Arkansas Polytechnic College at the age of sixteen. Nursing fed my soul, and I fell in love with critical care. Seeing so many people struggling with health issues strengthened my resolve to eat right, exercise the best I could, and learn about and do everything I could to be healthy. Relentlessly, I chased the dream of perfect health. Maybe that was why getting diagnosed with breast cancer shattered me to the core.

As a nurse since the age of nineteen, I thought I knew everything I needed to know about breast cancer. I understood treatment plans, surgical options of lumpectomies versus mastectomies, breast reconstruction, medications, and side effects, but nothing I learned as a nurse prepared me for the emotional devastation I experienced when I became a cancer patient. What I went through stunned me to an extent that I felt totally powerless in what was happening to my body, my life, or my mind.

I have a wickedly strong imagination so all the horrible possibilities of what *could* happen fueled by my nursing knowledge and experience flooded in to torment me constantly. Sleep was impossible and I wandered about my house in the middle of the night desperate for relief while trying not to wake anyone. Despite all my expertise, I still became a victim of fear.

One of the things I needed at the time was some kind of how-to book to understand what was happening, but I found nothing out there. There were inspirational stories of accomplishments like a cancer patient running marathons during chemo, but I felt I won a marathon when I made it to the toilet in time. Nothing spoke to me about how I was to get through all the disasters cancer brought into my life.

My cancer experience came before Facebook support groups were widely popular. I wasn't even on any social media at the time. Once I joined, I searched and found a few groups dedicated to breast cancer. But even with the community of other women with breast cancer that helped me not feel so alone anymore, there was something missing. I couldn't understand what was happening to me so I couldn't move forward, and I didn't feel like anyone around me really understood my challenges and struggles. I was paralyzed with fear, overwhelm, and indecision.

Realistically, there is no way to write the breast cancer self-help book I wanted because our experiences, prognoses, and treatment plans are so varied. A person at thirty has a different experience and set of needs than people in their sixties. However, there is one constant that all breast cancer patients share: loss. A diagnosis of breast cancer completely obliterates the life that was supposed to be.

In some form or measure, we all grapple with losses. Here, my nursing experience showed up to help me understand that what I was feeling was normal, even necessary, and giving myself permission to go through these emotions without judgment was healing. I hope that offering the framework of the grieving process will bring some comfort to anyone who is in the same position.

Loss brings grief and the grieving process in its wake. The American Psychological Association defines grief as the anguish experienced after a significant loss, usually the death of a beloved person, while the National Cancer Institute includes loss due to serious, long-term, or terminal illness. Most all definitions use a variety of terms that refer to strong, sometimes overwhelming emotions of sadness or despair.

It's normal to want to resist feeling any level of suffering but that will only prolong the pain and delay recovery. If we, instead, understand and appreciate how we need to grieve, seeing the process as normal and healing in its simplicity, it will guide us to understand and overcome our loss in an empowered way.

There are some myths and lies about grief that I experienced or heard from others which I feel hindered my process. They include the following:

❖ Grief is self pity.

❖ I don't have time to be sad.

❖ If I feel my sadness, it will only get worse.

❖ I am supposed to *only* think positively.

❖ If I acknowledge my grief, it will overwhelm me.

❖ I feel guilty I got cancer, so I am not entitled to feel sorry for myself.

All these became major stumbling blocks for me to feel and acknowledge my losses. They have a basic assumption that grief and the emotional chaos that happens is something overpowering, to be feared and avoided at all costs. My fear made my grief worse.

Grief is the natural reaction to loss of any kind. It is both personal and universal. Throughout my nursing career, I witnessed how any perceived loss could bring some measure of grief.

An accident or sudden life-altering illness meant changes, and those changes were always met with some form of grief because of the loss of what once was or at the very least, the loss of the dream of what *could* be. From something as simple as a lost set of keys or as devastating as death of a loved one, grief can be found. Loss is still very real even when it's for "good" reasons (like leaving a toxic relationship), because there is the absence of the future that was supposed to be (for example, one filled with intimacy and trust).

A diagnosis of cancer forever alters the trajectory of your life. It is something you cannot undo, hide from, or explain away—you can't fix it. Suddenly, you are on a roller coaster ride you didn't want to be on. A cancer diagnosis can be isolating, bringing fears of death, mutilation, pain, and loss in many forms, like jobs or careers, relationships, the ability to care for others, or financial stability. For some, a cancer diagnosis brings threats to body image, sexuality, or physical abilities. And the list goes on.

Perhaps you remember a time when you felt indestructible and confident in your good health. A cancer diagnosis shatters this and grief of all that will never be takes over. But it doesn't have to be that way; we can choose how we want to experience and process these unwanted, uninvited, and unwelcome changes, thereby taking back control in how we choose to experience and process these changes.

In 1989, Dr. Kenneth J. Dora coined a term, *disenfranchised grief*. This is where some forms of grief are not acknowledged by society as being significant and it is, therefore, dismissed. An example is when a person is told after a mastectomy with reconstruction, "At least you got a free boob job." The breast cancer veteran may not feel entitled to their grief around losing their breasts.

There is also some stigma around grief and grieving. It's socially okay to grieve as long as it is done for a specified amount of time or in a particular way. We are encouraged to get over it, get through it, get around it, stuff it down, think of others, ignore it, imagine it away—anything but acknowledge what we are feeling. Or sometimes, we are given specific rules for how we should handle, manage, or demonstrate our grief—anything but give ourselves permission to experience grief the way we need. Instead, if we would recognize and understand the overwhelming emotions as normal and even necessary in our healing from loss, it's possible that we could weather our grief with grace.

Elizabeth Kübler-Ross, a Swiss-American psychologist and pioneer in near-death studies, first introduced her five stages of grief model in her book *On Death and Dying* (1969) to help explain the emotional processes of coping with dying and loss. It has been greatly misunderstood as being linear and predictable, a rigid method that all people go through during grief. However, in later writings, Kübler-Ross revised her work to state that not all people go through all the emotional stages and perhaps not in any particular order or flow. However, in my practice as a nurse, I have never seen people skipping any of the phases entirely. Some appear to go through a phase in the blink of an eye without realizing they felt that stage at all, but they will, nevertheless, go through it.

According to David Kessler, who coauthored other books with Kübler-Ross, the model was never intended to wrap up messy emotions into neat little socially acceptable packages. Nor are they meant to be so systematic that we finish one stage, pass some symbolic test, and move on to the next level never to repeat the one before. These stages, or phases as I like to call them, may be thought of as fluid transitions through the emotional challenges that can come any time we experience grief. The depth, degree, intensity, or time required to process grief varies between individuals, but the methods are the same. Overall, the five stages of grief may be considered as a gentle guideline to frame and identify what is possible when experiencing grief. Others have adapted her initial work to include other stages or phases but for the purposes of this book, I'm sticking to the original framework by Kübler-Ross.

It is my hope that you can see how the acceptance of yourself at whatever phase you are dealing with is a way to bring healing into your life. Fighting this natural process of grieving your shock and trauma of getting a cancer diagnosis keeps you mired in places you don't want to be. I hope you are able to learn from my mistakes and laugh at the weird places my mind can go. My odd humor is my coping mechanism, so this book is an irreverent combination of my medical-provider input and a blatantly vulnerable look through my eyes at what I experienced as a patient.

You may note when reading that I avoid the label "breast cancer survivor". Not many people like to be lumped under identifying labels. In fact, the term *label* brings a level of resistance as if it is shoving us into categories limiting our potential. It smacks of exclusions and boundaries. However, labels can have a positive side and purpose. They help to identify a group by using a few descriptors. The breast cancer survivor label is exclusive to those who experienced but have not died as a result of breast cancer. It may also give a sense of community and lessen the sense of isolation that cancer brings.

According to the American Cancer Society's website from January of 2023, the breast cancer survivor label today represents somewhere around 3.8 million people in the US alone.

In writing this, I use the term *people* rather than women. Men can get breast cancer, also, which must be incredibly isolating when everything is directed toward the female gender. Breast cancer among men is rare but the few who are impacted have little community support.

Speaking of genders, that is a label that many are rebelling against in several ways. Our trans community or anyone who does not identify with gender labels can struggle to feel included as the literature speaks to women for the most part. Addressing someone as a "breast cancer sister" may intend to show communal support, but it can have quite the opposite effect.

For some, labels serve as inspiration and encouragement. For example, when I went through my cancer treatment, I liked to focus on *survivor* because it reminded me I was alive and fighting. I knew I had good odds of surviving, so I focused on that instead of on the possibility of treatment failure or reoccurrence. Then I focused on *warrior,* which reminded me to keep fighting and winning one battle at a time.

As time passed, daily life morphed. I came to terms with the fact that life would never go back to the *way it was* and I adjusted to the forced changes of the *way it is.* For me, breast cancer itself wasn't the hardest part. I never had pain or even felt the lump. It was the treatment and surgeries that devastated my world. Time has softened the memories, but I will never forget my experience. The personal growth I achieved as a result made me feel I was no longer *just* a survivor.

At one point as a result of my battle with cancer, I experienced what I felt was post-traumatic stress disorder (PTSD), so I looked up articles about PTSD and veterans. The more I read, a parallel showed up. The broad definition of *veteran* is a person who has long experience in a particular field. That describes me because I have long experience with breast cancer from both a medical and personal side. I feel I went through war myself, though my enemy was a faceless evil that threatened my very existence. I lost body parts and have multiple scars telling the story of my battles. Military veterans had no control of where they were sent or how they were to serve and neither did I. Yes, I could choose a unilateral or bilateral mastectomy with reconstruction as a possibility, but ultimately, I had to rely on the training and wisdom of others for my survival. Yet, I had no choice but to fight like hell.

Military veterans receive the label of veteran no matter how they served, whether on the front line or behind a desk. That feels more inclusive of people going through breast cancer from those with Stage 4 with metastasis to those with ductal carcinoma in situ (DCIS), which can require removal of the area and little else. I've known people who felt foolish to say they are breast cancer survivors because it wasn't as invasive as others. They experienced the very real trauma of receiving a breast cancer diagnosis so they should have their experience acknowledged also.

Being a military veteran comes with a measure of honor for their service and sacrifice, despite the role they played that a cancer survivor does not receive. It is easy to feel we have failed in some way to have gotten breast cancer. However, although none of us chose to get breast cancer, we do have the choice about how we respond to the losses that cancer creates in our lives. We choose how to serve and care for our loved ones, family, careers, and relationships. That alone is deserving of great honor.

Last but most importantly, PTSD in people who experience breast cancer is real and must be addressed to ensure the health and well-being of anyone who goes through it. Survival rates and health outcomes depend on more than just our medical treatment. Our mental and emotional health need attention and respect just as much as our physical bodies. Our lives mean so much more than just our survival.

The label of breast cancer survivor did so much for me when I needed it, but a time came when it wasn't big enough. I am so much more than merely alive. I am a breast cancer veteran.

For those who are not breast cancer veterans, I hope you are able to see through my experiences something about what breast cancer can do to a person's life. Whether you are a BC veteran or not, if you find yourself guilty of making any of the mistakes I present in this book, I hope you give yourself the grace to be human. This life is a learning field, not a test we have to ace to survive. Welcome to my story.

If Cancer is a Gift, Can I Return It?

This Can't Be Happening:
Shock and Denial

*Denial is the shock absorber for the soul. It
protects us until we are equipped to cope with
reality.*

C.S. Lewis

I'm sorry, it's cancer." According to the American Cancer
Society, Key Statistics for Breast Cancer, one in eight, or about
thirteen percent of women in the United States will hear those
words as I did. What many don't realize is that just hearing those
four words is traumatic in itself. They are an arrangement of words
that are life-altering and, more importantly, life-threatening. For
that reason, the mental and emotional health of a person diagnosed
with breast cancer must be addressed with as much respect and
care as their physical body. Too many people's lives are blasted by
cancer, and they are left floundering, trying to understand and
manage alone the devastation of cancer.

It's terrifying how four simple words become a wrecking ball
crashing through your life. You are not the same person you were
anymore. Now, you are someone facing cancer and all the scary
possibilities that having and treating cancer could bring. It's really
too much to take in at once. That's when shock and denial become
your best friends.

Anytime our brains register we are in danger, like getting
diagnosed with cancer because it ranks high on the list in life-

13

threatening experiences, the sympathetic nervous system, a primal portion of our brain, or the "lizard brain," jumps in to do its job. Its function is to trigger the biological changes for the fight, flight, or freeze reactions. It's because of these reactions that the prefrontal cortex (where reasoning, problem-solving, comprehension, and creativity are key) goes offline. Our lizard brains are pure self-protection and when activated, it is impossible to make well-thought out and rational decisions.

If your diagnosis came as a shock, the protective "freeze" reaction probably kicked in like a mental pause button until you could think again. It doesn't matter if we are facing a lion showdown or if we just heard shocking news, the process and effects of lizard brain are the same. We go into fight, flight, or freeze as a reaction to the stress. This makes it nearly impossible to take in and process whatever comes after hearing the word *cancer*.

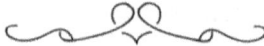

My appointment with my breast surgeon was early in the morning and she told me she would call me at the end of the day with the results of my biopsy. I went home feeling uneasy, but I didn't want to give up hope that everything would turn out okay. I wasn't going to allow negative thoughts to take over because that might make them come true. A part of me knew I was being silly, but I couldn't help myself.

It was close to five o'clock in the evening when the phone rang. Caller ID showed a number with the area code of my doctor, so I reluctantly answered it with a small "Hello?" I recognized the voice of my breast surgeon when she asked if I was Agalia Baker. I confirmed she had the right person.

"I'm sorry, it's cancer."

No, my brain said quite clearly. She's got this wrong. I don't have cancer. I can't have cancer. They screwed up somewhere. I refuse to have cancer. *Her words, as compassionate as they were, rattled around in my head failing to make any sense. I figured she was waiting for me to respond but my voice was frozen. My brain cells weren't speaking to each other enough to form a thought, much less a sentence.*

I finally said okay with zero emotion or affect because I was officially in shock. My brain was definitely offline and there were no signs it was rebooting anytime soon. She hesitated to speak but had to break the silence and tell me to come in so we would get a plan of what needed to be done. Still with no emotion, I said I would be there and hung up.

First, I called up my best friend and robotically informed her I had breast cancer and that I didn't want to talk about it. I hung up before she could say a word. If we still had the old-time landline phones, I would have slammed the receiver down. Then, I called my work nursing supervisor who knew about my having a suspicious lump. The call started out pretty calm and informative and then rapidly fell apart with my sobbing and screaming that I couldn't do this. "This can't be happening to me!" It probably would have been better if I had my meltdown with my bestie rather than my boss, but I don't do typical well.

A common reaction to getting a cancer diagnosis is to not believe what you are hearing. *Cancer can't happen to me. They got it wrong. They have the wrong chart, person, or test result.* It all has to be one huge mistake. Denial here is a comforting buffer to soften the blow until you have a chance to fully absorb what is being said. Some like me go numb, feeling nothing whatsoever.

My doctor could have been talking about the weather for all the impact it had on me. I couldn't handle it and my brain shut down.

It's also very normal to only be able to hear parts of what is being said. Your brain may just allow bits of information to get through leaving huge gaps between what you hear and what your medical provider *thinks* you hear. This is why you may need a lot of repetition before it all sinks in and a great reason to take someone along for the appointments.

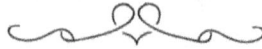

After I finished having my panic meltdown on the phone with my boss, I beelined for the one thing that helped me survive any stress in my life... my pool. I never knew how much I loved water because up to this point in my life, being around water only meant watching kids to make sure they didn't drown. When I moved to my dream home, I finally had a pool of my own. It became my liquid Xanax. No matter how stressful my day was, diving into the crystalline water would erase all my stress.

The partial lumpectomy and biopsy earlier that day was stressful enough but getting the results and screaming at my boss in a total emotional meltdown put my stress level over the top. I barely had my swimsuit on before I was out the door and standing on the diving board. My perfectly executed dive was exhilarating right up to the point that it felt like a mule kicked my left breast. Apparently, diving wasn't a good idea after having my breast gouged for a biopsy. Limping out of the pool clutching my aching breast, I felt like an idiot. Even though it was a stupid thing to do, I needed, for at least one moment, to forget I had cancer.

No matter how you react, now is not the time to beat yourself up for not thinking straight. My surgeon was pretty exasperated with me for diving in my pool after my biopsy because I could have really hurt myself. I should have and did know better. However, all my training, knowledge, and nursing expertise didn't keep me from blindly gravitating to something I knew made me feel better in the past.

Seeking Help from Others

Early days of a diagnosis can make you feel incredibly vulnerable. Some people prefer to reach out to others for help while others don't. One way is not better than the other. Just choose what feels right for you. We all need the space to do whatever is best for us without judgment and with the maximum support of our family, friends, and medical providers. Some people need to talk about their diagnosis over and over in an effort to help it sink in, perhaps even putting it out on social media while others must keep very quiet and private.

Going public in a format like social media isn't a good or bad thing to do but timing is important in making this decision. While in shock and denial to any degree, logical thinking is too difficult, and emotions are typically running high causing you to react in ways you wouldn't normally. This is not the best time to be making decisions with long-lasting effects like posting your cancer diagnosis or like in my case, screaming at a supervisor. Once you go public, you can't take it back, leaving yourself open to whatever reactions people have to your news. You may be someone who needs group support and social media can bring that, while at the same time, it can also cause people to distance themselves from you if they are unable to handle what you are going through. People distancing from you at a time like this is common, but it hurts. It's about them and their limitations, not you.

Going public also brings a tsunami of "advice" of which there will be some good and some really bad. Everyone has an opinion, and many are more than willing to tell you what you should do. It gets overwhelming and so very confusing. Right out of the starting gate I was told by one friend to do everything the doctor says, while another told me to refuse all medical treatments. As it turned out, I shouldn't have done everything the doctor said without question, but refusing all treatment could have meant my life. Having so many people telling me what I should do, feel, believe, or think was mentally taxing and contributed to the feeling of overwhelm.

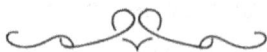

I realized I was a bit out of control with oversharing when I was standing at the bank counter talking to the teller, a young woman I've never met before, telling her all about my cancer and asking what she thought I should do about having a mastectomy. Not my finest moment.

The first few weeks after my diagnosis were harder for me. It seemed I was telling so many people for the first time about my cancer. Since I worked in several different clinics, I had a more than usual number of people who wanted or needed to know what was happening to me. Every time I told someone for the first time, I would see the shock in their eyes which reminded me how awful being diagnosed with cancer is. Sometimes I overshared like a garbage dump on people, and sometimes I could only give the basic facts. Ignoring cancer to feel somewhat normal for a little while was impossible since I had to talk about it all the time. If you find yourself doing as I, oversharing then regretting having to tell yet another person about your cancer, it's going to be okay. There are no rules here. Beyond the people in your work or personal life who need to be informed, you don't owe anyone anything more than what you feel like sharing at the moment.

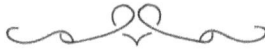

After my horrible phone call, the next few days were a blur. I saw my breast surgeon who told me I didn't have much choice, my breast had to come off. Then due to a misguided policy that has since been revised, I had a same-day appointment to see a plastic surgeon for reconstruction. I'm glad for the people coming behind me in this nightmare who do not have same day appointments. It's really too much too quickly.

The office of the plastic surgeon mailed me a packet of information and forms about the upcoming first stage of reconstructive surgery following the mastectomy. Only, the packet was delivered to my next-door neighbor I barely knew. Standing at my backyard picket fence, I saw her excitedly coming toward me waving a large manila envelope.

She handed me the envelope which had the plastic surgeon's office name and return address boldly printed in the corner. She started telling me she noticed I was going to have some plastic surgery and she wanted to let me know that she recommended a different surgeon because she had a tummy tuck which turned out so well. I struggled to know what to say or if I should just let her assume I was getting enhancements. She might ask me about it again later, so I opted for honesty.

I gently interrupted her and told her I had breast cancer. Her mouth dropped open, and I saw the flash of her unspoken thoughts shoot across her eyes. OMG! What have I stepped into? How could I be so stupid? How do I get out of this? Is there a hole nearby that I can be swallowed into? Oh, I'm making this about me, what should I say to Agalia? Then, out loud, she said, "Oh, I am so sorry."

I really felt sorry for her. My having cancer never dawned on her, and she was not an uncaring person. It was unfortunate, but I was put into the place of either reassuring her that it was okay or watching her flail about trying to pull her feet out of her mouth. It's not in my wheelhouse to let people suffer, so I reassured her with assurances I didn't have to give. She mumbled some other platitudes and scooted away quickly. Watching her go, it hit me...

What? She thinks I need a tummy tuck!

———————

Since denial is a protective coping mechanism that is very useful and necessary initially, give yourself all the time you need to work through all the emotions and fears you are dealing with. Let the awareness in a little at a time if you need to. This is the time to give yourself some kindness. Don't be surprised if you find yourself initially irritated with having to go through biopsies and repeated visits for further exams. You may think you don't have the time for this nonsense; there is too much to get done. *There are too many people relying on me. I don't have the time to do this now. I have to work. I have kids...*

Seeking Information

As unique individuals, we have a varied approach to challenges. Some find comfort in learning everything they can about the type of cancer, prognosis, treatment, and management. For others, avoiding learning anything beyond what is coming next is a way to put off what is happening. For them, the more you know, the more real it becomes. Caregivers for cancer veterans can get frustrated with the refusal to get informed about the cancer and treatment. However, it's okay to bury your head in the sand a little bit during this phase.

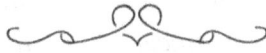

When I was a kid, I loved to read anything I could get my hands on. My reading speed was like lightning as I stopped seeing words and became a living part of the story. I could have sworn I heard thunder and smelled falling rain only to be confused when I came back to Earth and dry skies. Books were my escape. I could be anyone, anything, and anywhere I wanted to be between the pages of a book.

One day, I came across a book about a boy about my age, nine years old. He was from an abusive home and he, too, needed an escape. He taught himself to lean his head against a painting of an idyllic meadow scene complete with a small pond and swimming duck. He would put himself into a trance-like daydream where he was safe and contented. Sounded pretty great to me and I thought, I could do that too. So I tried it.

Turns out I was really good at dissociation. It was easy to slip away in my mind to the wonderful worlds of my imagination. Typically, I became some kind of superhero and saved everyone from evil without breaking a sweat. Sitting in classes or riding the bus, I was a million miles away. My brother was the reason I got off at the right stop or I would have gone home with the bus every day. I was that out of it.

To me, there was no downside to my trance-like daydreaming. It was everything I needed to feel safe, entertained, and happy. No way was I giving that up. As I became an adult, it got a little harder to completely shut out the world and my dream world faded quietly.

When I was diagnosed with breast cancer, I pulled out those dissociative skills and slipped into my identity as a nurse. I got really analytical and studied everything I could about my breast cancer. It was like it was happening to my patient, not me. I had planted a barrier between what was happening to me and what I allowed myself to feel. Only I couldn't sustain the distance as too much was crowding in, forcing me back into my real life, into my body. Dissociating as a kid was how I survived my childhood, but as an adult, it made getting through the phase of denial even tougher. I needed a little break from breast cancer, and that was the only way I knew how to get it. It just wasn't sustainable.

Total Denial

The danger of denial is that some may take it to extremes, refusing to accept the unwelcome news and therefore refusing to seek treatment. Some people can be in denial so strongly they convince themselves they really don't have cancer or that their illness isn't cancer at all. Others can deny the seriousness to the point that they refuse to follow up with a doctor about their diagnosis or seek treatment. To be clear, I am not talking about a person taking time to decide for themselves what action they want to take. Refusing to follow standard medical protocol is not necessarily pathological denial as long as you are making some kind of plan.

Total denial is the complete rejection of the significance or presence of cancer, not how you choose to address it. At this level of denial, one is pretending the cancer does not exist or even if it does, it has no bearing on their health or future. If you or someone you love is struggling with these types of reactions, professional help can be vitally necessary to getting well. Thankfully, this extreme denial is rare, and even prolonged common levels of denial don't happen that often. Once the cancer diagnosis has been accepted, denial in its initial intensity doesn't typically return.

As the initial shock fades, the lizard brain remains in control sending hormones, such as adrenaline, throughout the body to help you to fight or run from danger. Adrenaline helps the body to react quickly to a threat by making the heartbeat faster, increasing blood flow to muscles and the brain, and increasing blood sugar for fuel. This adrenaline rush gives you the energy to power through danger and an increased pain tolerance but can become a problem if activated too long or too frequently. The effects of an adrenaline rush can become a momentary crutch or addiction when relied upon too much. Here is a list of some things people may do to get an adrenaline rush to forget their pain for a few moments:

❖ Driving unsafely

❖ Unsafe sex

❖ Starting extreme sports such as skydiving, rock climbing, motorcycle racing

❖ Gambling

❖ Stealing

❖ Lying

❖ Drugs, alcohol

❖ Picking fights or arguing

❖ Debating controversial issues

❖ Eating disorders

Alcohol and drugs are probably more easily obtained and the more commonly used unhealthy options for dealing with the stress of cancer. They numb the emotional distress and pain, effectively allowing a moment to forget what you are going through. With chemo, however, alcohol may not be palatable due to the changes in taste. It also puts too much stress on the liver, which is burdened with eliminating the chemotherapy drugs. Additionally, alcohol worsens the side effects of chemotherapy and can cause dehydration, nausea, and mouth sores.

Another attempt to manage pain may show up as using food or over-exercising and the "feel-good" endorphins that are released to calm anxiety. Eating disorders such as anorexia, binge eating, and bulimia also give a false sense of control over your body.

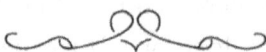

Shortly after my diagnosis, I was having lunch with my coworkers. I looked down at my healthy grilled chicken salad and my heart sank. It had felt like I'd controlled my diet forever and to what good? It was kind of embarrassing to have been a notorious food snob who got breast cancer.

"I should have ordered the fries and lived a little," I told them. One pushed her fries over to me, so I took one. It tasted like crap. All I could taste was old grease and salt and I hadn't even started chemo yet. Great. I finally decided to go rebel and the fries were awful. My belly voiced some displeasure, and I pushed them back. I'd stick with healthy eating even if my salad tasted like sawdust. My food snobbery didn't keep me from getting cancer but maybe I would feel the best I could until I found out how this cancer trip turned out.

A breast cancer diagnosis feels like it has stolen control of your life and future, so it is very normal to try to find a measure of personal control to combat the feelings of helplessness. If any of these words resonate with you, know that you are not broken. You are not alone. Please talk to your doctor or health care professional.

Don't stay silent in shame or hoping it will go away without help. You deserve better.

During my struggle with denial, I worked hard to stay busy, doing anything I could to not think about what was going to happen to me. I learned from the temporary insanity of my diving into the pool after my biopsy and the purple, bruised boob I got for my efforts. However, it is easy to take denial a little too far for safety. If this is you, I sincerely caution you to take care of yourself.

When Others Are in Denial

We generally think about how denial affects us when we get our cancer diagnosis, but it can show up in others, too. Family and friends get traumatized hearing your diagnosis and go into their own grieving and healing process. Even though it is not on the same level as your trauma and this is the time you need help from them the most, they may not be able to be there for you. It's frustrating that this is the hardest battle of your life and others are making your illness all about themselves. A parent may not be able to deal with the fact that their adult child is facing a life-threatening illness. A family member may feel you are creating this as a ploy for attention. A partner may not be able to face the sudden shift in responsibilities in the relationship. It's not fair but it happens.

Signs that others are in denial may include the following:

❖ They refuse to let you talk about your situation.

❖ They change the subject when you try to talk about what you are going through.

❖ They try to dismiss the fact that you are ill.

❖ They seem to ignore the fact that you have cancer.

❖ They downplay your anxiety, symptoms, or problems.

❖ They may be too busy to help when you need it.

❖ They may distance themselves from you.

People who react in these ways may be frightened about cancer themselves and are unable to deal with the emotions and fears that come up when they see you, especially if they have unresolved trauma that involved cancer. If they don't talk about it, they can pretend it's not real.

When dealing with someone in denial over your situation, the most important thing to do is to remember you need to take care of yourself first. It isn't generally helpful to confront or try to force the person in denial to acknowledge what you are going through. Trying to get the help or support you desperately need from a person in denial is a futile waste of your valuable energy. Gravitate to those who are able and willing to help or give you what you need.

Even though it is tough and grossly unfair, empathizing with them is necessary. Let them know you understand it is frightening for them to face what is happening to you but you need them by your side. Let them know how you feel. If they aren't taking your diagnosis seriously enough, let them know it hurts you for them to downplay your situation or experiences.

Dealing with people in denial about your cancer is especially difficult when they are close family members or friends. Realizing you can't rely on them at one of the lowest points in your life is devastating. Although understanding what they are going through is their own grief process and is not personal to you, the awareness that they aren't there for you is another loss you have to process within yourself.

Unfortunately, there are trolls who do exist and surface at the worst times. These are the people who insist you are lying to get more attention, sympathy, money, days off, an excuse to not do what they are having to do, and more. There have been those who have faked cancer for these reasons, but you do not need to explain or justify yourself to a troll. They can't hear you anyway.

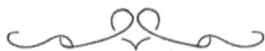

All trolls do not hide in the woods or under bridges. Some even look fairly human. A friend came to me after she had announced to her family that she was just diagnosed with breast cancer. Her sister (a.k.a. troll), with whom she had a rocky relationship, immediately got in her face, screaming that my friend was lying. The troll went on to insist my friend was only faking it to get attention and it wasn't going to work. She demanded to be allowed to talk to the oncologist and if my friend refused, it was proof that she was indeed lying about having cancer. Not only was my friend devastated by breast cancer, but she was also having to deal with the toxic waste dump that was her sister.

Transitions to the Next Phase

The trauma of shock and denial usually passes quickly, but there are some changes that make this initial period extremely problematic which are not necessarily a part of the grief process. As the freeze of shock fades, lizard brain is still on the job, flooding the body with stress hormones preparing you to be able to fight or run. Stress hormones make your heart pound; blood is diverted from organs to muscles to give extra strength, and non-essential body functions such as digestion are paused. Only, this isn't a lion, it is a cancer diagnosis, and there isn't anything tangible to hit or run from. Lizard brain doesn't know the difference. It is a purely biological component of the brain devoid of thought processes. It is there solely for your protection and to ensure your survival. You can't control it any more than you can continue to hold your breath after you pass out. Since it is a biological reaction and not a thought process, it is neither something a person should judge themselves about nor be judged for.

The stress hormones the lizard brain sends out trigger another part of the brain (the limbic system) where we process emotions, memories, and relationships. This portion of the brain uses past knowledge and experiences stored in emotional reactions or conditioning to provide information that can help predict the future. In other words, the lizard brain triggers fears.

If facing a lion, the body gets geared up to fight or run, and this portion of the brain pulls up all the past experiences or knowledge about lions for the best survival tactics. Where lizard brain is instinctive, this section is intuitive information and fears. The purpose is to bring anything that you have experienced in the past around the danger you are presented with to give you clues as to what to do or expect. Past experiences and knowledge about breast cancer influence greatly how intense the fears are. Then fears evolve around how well you were supported in the past, about your work or job status, family's needs, what impact it will have on your partner or your relationships, just to name a few.

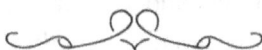

When I was first diagnosed, my supervisor offered me extra time off and I took it. Big mistake. On one hand, my job responsibilities required me to be fully present and my clients deserved that. It was a bonus to them to not have me there going through the motions of providing medical care while my brain was officially checked out of commission.

On the other hand, time off was sheer hell. It gave me way too much time to think or more accurately, try not to think. I tormented myself with relentless questions about what I did so wrong that I got breast cancer, whether I was choosing the best treatment options, and if, along with my breast, my life and marriage were going to be mutilated. By this time, I was reassured that my cancer hadn't spread to the lymph nodes which was good news. I wasn't afraid of dying of cancer because my brain wouldn't go there. Denial showed up for me in a pure form of not even considering that I might die. Living was hard enough.

After all this, I came to realize that ten minutes alone with my imagination was deemed cruel and unusual punishment.

Fear can feel like punishment for mistakes or wrong choices in the past, but it is simply a protective measure of the mind. All the fears I was experiencing after my diagnosis were perfectly normal attempts by my brain to inform me of potential outcomes and help me make the best decisions. It *felt* like absolute hell.

This is also a time when all the people who love someone experiencing cancer are also impacted with the anxiety and fears driven by their lizard brains. When everything is unknown, the entire future is in upheaval, fears of what *may* happen start to take over.

Seeking Calm after the Storm

Once danger has passed, the parasympathetic nervous system is there to help the body calm down and relax. However, stress of a cancer diagnosis continues relentlessly preventing the parasympathetic system from doing its job. Stress, tension, and its effects on our bodies become chronic, creating anxiety and keeping the sympathetic system on alert. The high levels of stress hormones like cortisol disrupt your sleep, make you reach for comfort food, and cause you to feel hypervigilant to danger from every angle. It's exhausting.

The extra energy created by stress hormones is meant to be used up quickly so the body can start to relax. When stress and anxiety can't be released, we have to do something to burn off the nervous energy. Pacing, being jittery, and bustling around doing mindless tasks are among the many ways the body tries to burn off these hormones and their influences. Some people laugh when nervous and if that is you, go with it. Releasing nervous energy is necessary. Fighting your natural inclinations prevents your body from relaxing and your hormone levels from returning to normal.

Focusing on calming, anxiety-reducing relaxation strategies will help you throughout your cancer journey. All the fears running through your mind keep your attention either in the past or the future, never in the present moment. Fear of past mistakes coming to light, or repeating themselves, keeps you ruminating on every move—every choice you've ever made—while fear of the future and whatever it will bring keeps you stressed, tense, and anxious. The key to relaxation is bringing your attention and focus to the present moment. It sounds simple but nothing could be further from the truth in a time while you're in it.

Relaxation releases tension, lowering blood pressure which increases blood circulation in the body. This brings more energy while helping you to have a calmer, clearer mind aiding in better memory, concentration, positive thinking, and improved decision-making skills. Most relaxation techniques aim to bring your attention to the present, giving your body a moment to unwind and be able to breathe.

Gentle massage and acupuncture may be an option for helping with stress relief.

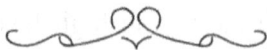

I got a gift certificate for a massage that I was happy to use. I checked with my doctor, got her blessings, and called to get my appointment. The therapist answered and just as soon as I told her my name, she coldly said, "You can't have a massage if you have breast cancer." This is

one of the problems of living in a small town. Everyone knows your business. First of all, since she was a stranger to me, the gift certificate benefactor must have been talking about me. Second, if she knew I had breast cancer, why did she sell them the gift certificate in the first place?

Not wanting to give up, I asked, "Why can't people who have breast cancer get massages?"

"I have rules to follow, and you can't have a massage if you have breast cancer."

"Can I get a refund on the cost of the gift certificate?"

"No." Her cold tone of voice frostbit the ear my phone was pressed to. This convo was making me feel more like I had leprosy rather than breast cancer. Being stuck with a gift certificate I wasn't going to be able to use was defeating, too. I didn't know what to do so I did the only thing I could. I lied.

"Well, it's a good thing I don't have breast cancer."

She didn't believe me, but she couldn't refuse me. By the way, the massage really sucked and didn't reduce any stress, but I got a little satisfaction in getting my way.

As with any complementary treatment, check with your oncologist or breast surgeon before adding something to your treatment protocol.

Whatever methods you choose, it is important to practice relaxation. Some prefer guided imagery, journaling, practicing gratitude, or sharing their experiences with family or friends. Others find it helps to seek a source of spiritual support or a counselor. Setting some time aside to be alone can be restoring. Be ready to say no to the things that cause you more stress. Now is the time to put yourself first. The techniques I list below are among some that I learned after the fact. I hope you don't do as I did and spend too much time tortured by anxiety. Here are a few practices I incorporated that helped me. None of this is one-size-fits-all, so try what you like and stick with what fits.

4-7-8 Breathing: Breathe in through your nose to a count of four, hold your breath for a count of seven then breathe out audibly through your mouth for a count of eight. When we are tense, we breathe shallowly which increases heart rate, blood pressure, and stress. Focusing on breathing keeps you present and distracted from negative thoughts and emotions. Try to breathe deeply, allowing your belly to expand and relax freely. Having a flat stomach is considered in several cultures to be more attractive but holding the stomach in is a common practice that inhibits deep breathing. For many, tense shallow breathing is so ingrained that breathing deeply feels unnatural.

Rule of 3-3-3: Look for three things you can see around you, then listen for three things you can hear, and then move three parts of your body (e.g., fingers, toes, shoulders). This is a grounding exercise that reduces stress by helping you focus on your environment therefore disrupting negative thought patterns. This is one that is easier to do without anyone else noticing what you are doing.

Attention Shift Between Inner and Outer Sensations: Shift your attention back and forth between inner and outer sensations. Focus on something outside of you such as something you can see or hear. Then focus on something you feel inside your body like the pressure of your butt in the chair or your unsettled stomach. Keep switching back and forth between the inner and outer sensations until you feel calmer. This exercise also helps you focus attention on the present and become more grounded. The benefit of this one is that it helps to focus on something in your environment and then something you feel in your body (somatic sensations). It helps to lessen dissociation to a small extent. Dissociation can make you feel disconnected from your body, thoughts, or emotions. Again, it's an attempt by the brain to protect you from stress but can hinder getting past the anxiety.

Being in Nature: Try going for a walk, gardening, walking outside with your bare feet, or hugging a tree. There is mounting evidence that being in nature lowers stress, improves attention, and elevates mood. If you can't be outside, research has shown that images or sounds of nature also give benefit. Houseplants, aquariums, and pets all are effective in reducing stress as long as you have the energy to care for them appropriately.

Exercise, Sports, and Water: Exercise and sports release endorphins helping you to feel better while being immersed in water stimulates the parasympathetic nervous system which is responsible for relaxation. Please check with your doctor about when it is safe to take baths or swim. Surgical sites, radiation burns, and broken skin need to be healed before soaking or swimming.

Finally, the Storm Does Ease

Only when your lizard brain is quieted is the logical, thinking portion or rational brain able to function smoothly. Rational brain is the portion of our brains where we are able to be self-aware, to think, analyze, and be reasonable. It is a quieter voice that is detached from emotions. Its purpose is to make sense of what is happening in our life and to make the best decisions for ourselves. Unfortunately, the lizard brain screams the loudest and the emotional part feels the strongest, making it nearly impossible for the rational brain to work efficiently when you are needing it most. It's like having three different voices with vastly different opinions in your head all trying to talk at the same time causing great confusion.

It's understandable that it is best to postpone any major decisions until you calm down but typically you don't get a chance to do so. Decisions such as treatment options, work, and childcare needs among others are forced upon you immediately, long before your rational brain can figure out what to do.

Denial in some form is natural, normal, and even necessary for our well-being. It is only when it goes too far that it can get problematic. Berating ourselves for reacting in shock and denial or trying to avoid the reality of cancer is how we get stuck in our healing. This is a time to be gentle with yourself. If you need to talk, reach out to someone, but if they can't give you what you need, don't take it personally. Find a professional or someone qualified to help you.

Social media groups and chat rooms serve a purpose of establishing community but don't necessarily give you the intense, individual attention you may want or need. You deserve to be able to ask for help. If you are more like me and don't want to talk about it twenty-four seven, that's okay too. This phase, too, shall pass.

Getting Pissed:
Anger

Where there is anger,
there is always pain underneath.

Eckhart Tolle

Anger really gets a bad rap. In the context of the grieving process and the aftereffects of shock, it's the natural process of our autonomic systems giving us the energy to fight back at whatever is threatening us. However, no other emotion is vilified as much as anger is. As women, we are more often taught that anger is not socially acceptable and that we must, above all, be nice. The pressure to hide anger seems to be lessening because an enormous number of people are willing to go ballistic these days. Or perhaps, suppressed anger has breached the emotional pressure valve and people just can't take any more injustices. Whatever the reason, it seems we have been taught that controlling anger is more important than addressing what is causing our anger.

Some cultural, religious, and societal norms stress restraint and demonize anger to keep people from killing each other. The intent is good but the extent to which people are compelled to resist anger is tremendous. Constantly suppressing anger only intensifies it to the point of loss of control and the emotional pressure value blows. Then society steps in to exert even more control, punishment, or negative consequences to subdue the people and the anger. Probably everyone on this planet has been on the receiving end of someone's uncontrolled anger. That can make anger and the repercussions of anger get embedded into our minds as something scary and to be avoided at all costs.

Anger is really telling us someone or something is violating our boundaries. It isn't evil in and of itself. It's what we choose to allow anger to make us do, say, or feel that gets dangerous.

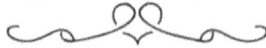

<hr>

Reality sank in. The sweet reprieve of shock and denial was wearing off and instinctual anger came rushing in. Being diagnosed with breast cancer felt like the ultimate betrayal by my own body. The temptation to lash out was so normal yet I judged myself and reined it in like anger was scarier than cancer. Just like a startled dog that blindly snaps and growls, I was flooded with an over-whelming desire to fight something. I just didn't know what. I felt powerless, overwhelmed, and terrified. Of course, I got angry. I didn't know who to blame, whether I should be lashing out at God, myself, or some other unknown entity for inventing the carcinogens that have polluted our environment and convinced me they were safe.

<hr>

As a woman born during the tail-end of the baby boomer generation, I was trained to keep a tight rein on my emotions—anger in particular. Displays of anger, no matter how justified, were specifically forbidden according to social norms of my time. There were rebels against this train of thought who were able to stand up to injustices, but I wasn't one of them.

In many cultures, women are put under intense pressure to conceal anger even to the point they don't recognize it in them-selves. Concealed or repressed anger has a short fuse that can be easily triggered and explode in the form of hurtful words or actions. Think of a stress squeeze ball as anger. The more we try to repress it by squeezing it tightly in our hands, the harder it works to bulge out in funky ways and directions. It tends to erupt wherever it can but not always where it is needed.

Anger is an emotion that doesn't always show up alone. Unlike happiness which is pretty straightforward, anger can hide behind sorrow or fear. Especially if you are a person who doesn't default to anger, sorrow can be what shows up predominantly. Sorrow is an emotion that is more socially and personally acceptable to express so the anger beneath the sorrow remains unnoticed and starts to fester. Conversely, anger covers up deep sadness and fears. Sometimes it's easier to get angry than to face the sadness and fear lurking deep within us.

If you think of cancer as a hurricane you are weathering, the emotion of anger can feel like a spin-off tornado of destruction within your personal hurricane. It comes with a mini cycle of grief on its own. Just like there are cycles in the grieving process around getting a cancer diagnosis, there are also cycles in dealing with the anger. The tendency is to deny your anger, get angry that you are in a situation that makes you angry, reason or bargain away your anger, and even get depressed when your anger doesn't feel like it accomplishes what you truly want. Since anger can feel so shameful, it's easy to beat yourself up for feeling it.

Anger is also harder to control when you are at your most vulnerable. When you are dealing with cancer, cancer treatment, and this grieving process, it is easy for things to set you off where they never would have bothered you before. Small infractions can feel intolerable. Anytime you don't feel well, it is difficult to operate at your highest capacity even though you may desperately want to do so. This is a time you may need, want, or expect more help from others. If your needs go unmet, it can be extremely frustrating. Venting your frustration can get complicated if whoever you are dealing with is unwilling or unable to meet your needs because your anger can make them even less receptive. You could be someone who hates to ask for help but silently wishes someone would notice. If they don't, it's easy to be angry at their inconsiderateness. It's important to ask for help when you need it before you get frustrated. If they are unwilling to give you what you need, at least you will know.

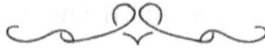

∽∾♡∾∽

Anger is danger. That's what I learned early in life. I grew up in an angry home and saw firsthand the damage unchecked anger does. Therein lies the distinction, unchecked anger. It's like in the Goldilocks story, anger can't be too hot or too cold. It has to be just right. Trouble is, I was trained that anger was wrong under any circumstances and never taught how to safely manage and release anger in a healthy way.

My mother seemed to thrive on anger, and she would pick fights with anyone just for the sake of fighting, which terrified me. I learned to avoid her whenever she was in one of her moods and hide in my bedroom. She would turn on anyone who crossed her path even if they had nothing to do with what she was upset about. I got really good at fading into the background whenever she was around like the alien in the movie Predator. Anything to avoid getting in her line of vision. I also learned I could never stand up to her or fight back because I could always be outclassed in the verbal defensive arts. In fact, everyone could "out anger" me. I had four older brothers, which is a lesson in futility in itself for winning an argument. I didn't fight the older ones, though. I wasn't stupid. Even my youngest brother could easily hold me at arm's length with his hand on my forehead as I windmilled my arms trying to land a blow on him. I learned to swallow all my emotions to survive and now people are telling me I got cancer because I was repressed. Seems it's a case of damned if you do, damned if you don't.

I grew up stuffing my feelings down. All of them, anger included. In his book, *The Body Keeps the Score*, Dr. Bessel van der Kolk states that emotions and trauma, in particular, if left unexpressed and unacknowledged, may become lodged, disruptive energy within the body. What I appreciated about his work was there was no blame, no judgment for having stuck energy. It is simply a fact that it happens and is a sign that many people need help to process their trauma.

Adverse childhood experiences (ACEs) are defined as potentially traumatic events that occur before a child turns eighteen years old. These events can affect a person's health, opportunities, and stability throughout their lifetime and possibly generations to come. Studies show the more ACEs a child suffers, the more likely they as adults will develop chronic health conditions, anxiety, or depression, and engage in risky behaviors which include smoking, substance abuse, and violence. It will come as no surprise to anyone that cancer is one of the health conditions listed. With all these factors, there is no way we can be judgmental with ourselves in how we have handled our lives so far. We can only accept ourselves as we are right now and pick up the pieces of our lives believing we are doing our best.

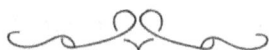

My childhood has an ACE score that's way up there. It's not something I take pride in. Nor do I really want to even think, much less write, about it. However, what I've experienced shaped my reactions to everything life has brought me. It took me plenty of years to learn that

carrying the burden of childhood trauma doesn't have to be a life sentence. There are ways to release that pain.

Of all my ACEs, profound physical and emotional neglect was and, in some ways, still is the hardest to shake. Physical abuse seems easier to bear because you at least are noticed. Everyone knows you don't hit kids, so you get a little more compassion from society. With neglect, it almost feels like you are being "too sensitive" or complaining about not getting enough attention, but it left me feeling like I could disappear off the face of the Earth and no one would notice.

Neglect during my childhood set me up to constantly try to prove myself valuable throughout my life. I became a people pleaser, trying to get people to like and accept me. I drove myself to be someone I wasn't just because I thought that was someone other people wanted.

Well beyond childhood, it felt like I had a "Kick Me" sign on my back because people seemed to think it was okay to do so. I thought that was what I deserved too. I never fought back, never stood up for myself, and no one stood up for me. After all, I was teaching people how to treat me by taking their abuse. Once cancer hit, I took it as a sign that everyone was right, I deserved what I got.

I should have gotten angry about how I was treated, but anger was too scary because of the violence I'd witnessed. My go-to reaction in the face of conflict was to freeze like a popsicle. I called it my fainting goat syndrome.

Because of cancer, I got tired of taking the blows and I slowly started standing up to people who either actively or passively hurt me. It wasn't okay anymore. I still didn't use anger, though. That's just not me. I did grow a few boundaries. I cut some toxic people out of my life and made room for good relationships. I stopped people pleasing and started believing in me. Even though I did not feel my worth, I chose to believe I had value simply because I exist.

If you think I got there overnight, you would be wrong. It took baby steps, the occasional panic attack, and a lot of hard work. Facing the crap we have dealt with in life without becoming victimized by it is excruciatingly difficult but so worth it. If you have to get pissed to take up for yourself, you have every right to do so.

There have been some older studies done on anger and cancer which apparently show a strong connection between repressing anger and ultimately being diagnosed with cancer. While the evidence shows a correlation between cancer and suppressed anger, it is important to not use this information as judgment of yourself. It is easy to think you did this to yourself. You may think that if you weren't the person you are or had you not repressed your anger over your lifetime, you wouldn't have gotten cancer. However or whatever you learned about anger and anger management since childhood shouldn't be used to beat yourself up. You may have done the best you could to survive at the time, but now you are free to do things differently.

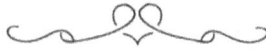

I was working in a health department and was between clients who were waiting for their exams and birth control. A nurse working with me walked up to me and said, "You know, cancer is anger turned inward."

I'm not one of those quick-witted people so I probably stood there with my mouth hanging open until she left. Are you kidding me? She didn't just tell me to my face that I got cancer because of some kind of character flaw! I gave this to myself for being too nice? Or is she saying I'm phony, that I act all sweet on the outside and I'm really a seething pus pocket of anger inside?

Implying to someone that they are in some way responsible for their getting cancer is one of the most hurtful, injurious things to do to them. The nurse who said that to me has every right to form her opinion as to why I got cancer, but I didn't ask her opinion. In fact, the blatant disregard for how it would make me feel is a violation that made me angry. Only it was too late. She was gone and I was left trying to repress my anger once again. No more. I've had a few years to think up a good comeback. I know what to say now. Bring it on, chickadee.

Cancer Is Not the Result of a Character Flaw

One of the most harmful problems with blame is it brings the word *should* into our lives. If cancer was my wake-up call to stop repressing anger, the natural flip side is that I should have not repressed my anger. Or, I should have learned how to manage my anger better or developed better boundaries. *Should* is an active form of self-criticism. "Shoulds" mean we don't accept ourselves for who and where we are. They cause us to reject ourselves and the choices we have made, which increases anxiety and stress. *Should* is a word that needs abolishing.

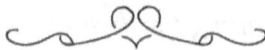

I follow a Facebook group created for those who chose to go "flat" (no reconstruction after mastectomies). It is made up of people who have either bilateral or unilateral mastectomies, and who chose to go straight to flat, and several who had expanders or implants removed. One

woman posted a plea for help when a member of her family voiced her inexcusably inconsiderate opinion. It highlighted the pain caused by insensitive words.

The woman wrote that she was facing a mastectomy and was talking to her son and daughter-in-law (a physician) about what she should do related to going flat or reconstruction. Her daughter-in-law spoke up and told her she should just get them cut off and forget it, but where she really messed up was to not have made lifestyle changes ten years ago. The daughter-in-law went on to claim that she needed to view her cancer as her "wake-up call."

The woman was devastated, shocked, and understandably angry. She wrote that she was torn between wanting to cry or bitch-slap her daughter-in-law. What stopped her was the fact that she had a new grandson and if she told her daughter-in-law how she felt, it could cost her a relationship with him. She held it together enough to get out of there but was seeking help with the butt-load of trauma the situation caused.

She went on to explain that she had stopped smoking years ago and although her diet wasn't pristine, she avoided trans fats and too much sugar. She was doubting herself and every decision she had ever made regarding her health. She asked for help of what to do or say to her son and daughter-in-law, or whether she should just let it go. The pain in her plea for help struck me to the core.

The responses she received were warm and compassionate with several coming to her defense using choice adjectives describing her daughter-in-law. Many wrote how they were super health conscious or athletic and still got cancer. A couple wrote a few snarky come-backs for the next time. (Sad, but true that there could be a next time.) Throughout all the support she received, there still wasn't a clear option of how to handle the trauma. The woman was suffering from the trauma of having cancer, having to decide how to approach it surgically but now she was faced with judgment from her family, fear of losing her grandson, and self-judgment to boot.

If she bitch-slapped her daughter-in-law, that might feel good for a minute, but the price may be her relationship with her son and grandson. It almost smacks of emotional blackmail to put up with someone's bad behavior simply because they can take so much away from you. Yet, it happens too many times. If she tried to debate with her daughter-in-law that healthy people get cancer too, it would just start a "right fight" where most likely, they will choose to die on the hill of their beliefs and there isn't a thing you can say that will change their minds. Her daughter-in-law is a doctor who should have known better anyway.

If she chose to not bring it up with her son and daughter-in-law, she runs the risk of stuffing her feelings down until they fester only to explode at a later date. Festering resentment poisons the one holding it. The offender gets off scot-free.

She sucks at snarky comebacks as I do. When I get blasted by heartless words, I freeze, my mind goes blank, and I am deer-in-the-headlights frozen solid. Any snark that comes to mind occurs no sooner than ten minutes past too late. My lizard brain goes straight to the freeze form of the fight/flight/freeze reaction. My next reaction is to run away like my tail feathers are on fire, which is the flight reaction. Some people instinctively lash out in anger which is the fight response. Apparently, the woman experienced all these types of reactivity of lizard brain at once and didn't know how to handle it.

Unfortunately, it's really hard to plan how to react because it depends on your most common instinct whether it's fight, flight, or freeze. It takes practice to respond—not react—in situations like this. For her, a little self-compassion is needed. She reacted instinctively in the moment and that's okay. That's the best anyone can do. She can't beat herself up for not engaging in a verbal debate on her health choices of the last ten years or that health activists get cancer too. She would have to deal with the fallout if she fought back. Had she bitch-slapped her daughter-in-law, her problems would be different from those of the flight or freeze reaction. If she never talks about her feelings to them, she will have to deal with the resentment that comes with silence.

I hope she comes to the realization that her daughter-in-law's words are a reflection of her daughter-in-law, not her, and beating herself up for past decisions and choices is useless and unnecessary. It will be great if one day, she is able to say in a non-emotionally charged voice, "I was shocked and hurt you would say those things to me whether they are true or not." Until that day, I hope she gives herself a break for being human, something her immature, insensitive, and ignorant daughter-in-law fails miserably at.

Yeah, I may have been one of those with lots of adjectives.

The ways anger shows up can be so varied. It is not always an initial reaction but can accumulate over a period of time. The more we see unaddressed injustices, the more fuel there is to stoke the fires of anger.

You might feel angry at:

❖ the people closest to you.

❖ feeling pressured to function normally at the expense of your health.

❖ the doctors and nurses or the entire health care system.

❖ the complexity and limitations of insurance systems.

❖ God, the Universe, or your spirituality or religious beliefs.

❖ people who are well while you are not.

❖ people who say or do insensitive things out of ignorance.

❖ the loss of the dream you hoped for your life.

❖ the loss of self-reliance and now needing help.

❖ the loss of your plans for your future.

❖ any changes or losses in relationships.

❖ any perceived changes in your identity or roles in your life.

❖ all the things I failed to include in this list.

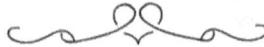

A couple of days after my mammogram that bombed, I was scheduled to see a breast surgeon for the first time. I was heart-pounding, gut-clenched scared. I took my knitting with me to soothe myself with something to do with my hands, which were in a blur of furious movement. Sitting for what felt like forever half naked in a tiny, airless room waiting for a harbinger of doom to come in, I was admittedly a bit tense.

A nurse came in to enter all my pertinent data and past medical history into the computer. Being in the medical field, I was familiar with all these questions and was prepared to answer and viciously knit at the same time. She started with the usual and I answered on autopilot until she got to my parental health history. My mother died in the eighties and to put it gently, I was not her favorite child by far. In fact, everyone else's child would make the list ahead of me.

The nurse asked about her medical history, and I replied that she passed due to metastatic cancer. She disinterestedly asked what kind and I said I didn't know.

For the first time, the nurse paused and turned her head to really look at me and said in the coldest voice possible, "Do you mean your mother died of cancer, and you don't know what kind?" The ice on that verbal knife was chilling.

A bit shocked, I sucked in a breath and said, "No, I was never told." Good thing I was knitting 100 percent cotton washcloths because I would have shredded yarn by then.

This joy of a nurse, still staring coldly at me over her shoulder said, "Well, it's important."

My first response was No shit, Sherlock. Did I say that out loud to this person who lacked a soul and needed to hear it? Of course not. I'm far too professional, far too NICE! I was trained to believe it is not safe to say what you really think, and I get green with envy over people who can. When I grow up, I'm going to be more like them.

I cry when I'm angry, but I refused to cry in front of this evil nurse from the bowels of hell, so I sucked it up and continued answering her questions. I barely remember anything the surgeon said when she came in. Before long, I was shuffled off to be poked and prodded by more medical equipment holding back my tears until my throat hurt.

The next day, I was going through my email, and lo and behold, I saw a survey of that office visit. The wicked smile of the Grinch Who Stole Christmas stretched across my face. Nurse Ratched was about to meet karma who could be a real bitch. Seriously though, people like that shouldn't be nurses much less in an oncology department. She might have been having a rough day and it was showing up as judgment, but her actions were inexcusable.

I just found out I had cancer, so I could relate to having a bad day. I have tons of knitted washcloths to prove it.

Healthy Anger

What is healthy anger anyway? One definition says something to the effect that it is observing and experiencing anger without being overwhelmed by it and reacting to it. To me, that sounds more like analytically separating yourself from the emotion of anger rather than acknowledging the anger felt and managing it in a positive way. True, the expression and release of anger needs to be done in a way that we don't do damage to others, ourselves, relationships, or anything that doesn't need to be destroyed. If you do an internet search on expressing anger in a healthy way, you find lists that suggest taking deep breaths, reciting mantras, doing visualization, and changing your surroundings, among others. These are fantastic ways to dismiss, disarm, and avoid anger so you don't actually have to feel it. These techniques may help your anger to not spiral out of control, which is important but not the entire solution.

It is commonly understood that holding anger in is bad for you. On the other hand, sudden outbursts or prolonged anger can be bad for you, too. Strong emotions such as anger can intensify the hormonal effects on the body, escalating the emotion until it is beyond control, leaving damaging effects in its wake. Chronic anger stimulates the reactive fight or flight of the lizard brain releasing cortisol and adrenaline. These hormones impact the body, raising the blood pressure and diverting blood flow away from the gut to the muscles in order to run from danger. If lizard brain stays activated, we become frozen in a self-protective state.

If our bodies are designed to be flooded with hormones that give us the energy and ability to fight an aggressor and get angry, then to put all the responsibility for management on our mental and emotional strength is, in my opinion, wrong. We may need to physically burn off those hormones in a healthy way. Some people need to run, put on boxing gloves and actually punch something, go in the bathroom and scream until their throats are raw, or beat a pillow to death. Anger power is animalistic and maybe that is what is so frightening. However, if we expect to deal with animalistic energy only with mental control and calculated physical measures, our anger can only be partially released. Using our thinking brains to control our emotions does not process and release anger the way we have been trained to believe.

By finding appropriate and healthy ways to release anger, we avoid taking it out on everyone around us. Suppressed anger shows up as irritability, having a short fuse, impatience, frustration, passive aggression, and saying or doing things that ultimately make us feel worse about ourselves. Most of all, by accepting our need and right to move anger out of our bodies, the anger will not get so unmanageable in the first place.

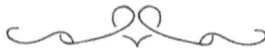

Right now, I wish I were writing a bit about how I did such a fantastic job of displaying healthy anger management. I can't because I didn't. I managed to make my way through this entire part of my life without breaking form. I never told people who upset me what I felt, nor did I ever raise my voice, break dishes, throw stuff, or anything else I advise you to do. My little companion dog, Maggie, is

partially the reason. If I ever raised my voice, she would cower, and I felt like an ogre. I could scowl at her, and she shook in fear that she was about to be whipped. I never hit her, but because she was a rescue, there's no telling where she learned about anger.

Having the kindest husband with the patience of Job really helped. He never has been an angry person and honestly models healthy anger management. He isn't a pushover but has a long, slow fuse and blastoff has only happened a few times since I've known him. Fighting sometimes happened when we were young and dumb but hasn't been a factor in our marriage for many years.

The last time we disagreed, for some reason unknown to humankind, instead of my bickering, I said, "It hurt my feelings when you said that."

He looked a bit startled and replied, "I didn't mean to hurt your feelings." He told me then how he felt, and we worked it out.

Somewhere in the passage of time, I learned to not be such a people pleaser. That was how I survived before, but it doesn't suit me now. I've learned that I don't have to justify my feelings or reasons to anyone unless I want to. I have every right to state how I feel and not be responsible for how the other feels about it. Unless, of course, I tack judgment on the end like, "It hurt my feelings when..., you jerk."

Anger Affects Others

People around you probably don't know how to deal with your anger. The common theme is that they tend to take it personally, creating more drama and pressure to soothe their feelings when yours are still out of control. Informing your family and loved ones what is happening is important. Telling a child mommy is angry at cancer but not them helps. Explaining that mommy is "going in the other room to scream really loudly at cancer" enables them to understand that it isn't their fault you are angry. Telling them you will be okay and after you have "screamed at cancer enough," you will "be back and will feel much better" helps them to know there is an expected end to the unstable emotions they are sensing. Modeling appropriate anger management to others will help change the stigma around anger as well as redefine what healthy anger is.

We need a clear understanding of the value and purpose of anger to appropriately manage it. As long as we consider anger unacceptable, we stay in a state of arousal that prevents us from being able to regulate our thoughts and behaviors, staying focused only on our inner emotional state. Believing all anger is bad keeps you from feeling you have a right to be angry or to stand up for yourself. Recognizing the positive aspects of anger helps us to identify and label what we are feeling and why. If we can focus on why we are angry instead of the judgments of feeling the anger, we won't feel as powerless to use the motivations of anger in a positive way.

The Good Side of Anger

There are some upsides to anger that aren't as mainstream as they should be. However, there is more being written by social and evolutionary psychologists and mental health professionals suggesting anger has valuable benefits. All emotions are appropriate when experienced at an optimal level, meaning that the Goldilocks theory of *just right* is important. Repressed emotions are "too cold" and not processed in a healthy way. You have to allow yourself to feel an emotion to address it. On the other end of the spectrum, being uncontrollably engulfed in an emotion is "too hot" or potentially damaging. Somewhere in the middle is ideal. Emotions are acknowledged and felt but remain in a zone of manageability. Just as sadness can elicit appreciation for what we have lost, stress can enhance performance, and mild anger can help us to move forward with better understanding of ourselves and what we need.

In writing this section, I had to do a massive amount of research to understand the ins and outs of anger. Thankfully, I ran across several articles and blogs that spoke to possible positive sides to anger which were very intriguing concepts. Compiling the basic concepts helped me to look at anger differently, as something not quite so shameful but in fact, potentially useful in some situations.

- ❖ **Anger is a survival tool.** It is deeply embedded in our primal need for survival and protection from aggression and is the energy to push back and fight when we need to.

- ❖ **Anger provides a sense of control.** It helps us to protect what is ours or what is happening to us rather than feeling helpless and victimized by others or situations. A word of caution is to not become obsessed with the sense of power that anger brings.

- ❖ **Anger is motivational.** It gives us a stimulus to find solutions or make changes to resolve our problems.

- ❖ **Anger highlights injustice.** It is an internal guidance system that tells us something is wrong with the way we or others are being treated.

- ❖ **Anger keeps us focused upon our goals.** It pushes us toward achieving our goals and ideals.

- ❖ **Anger triggers hope.** It keeps us focused on what we hope to attain instead of the pain, insult, or victimization of a situation. Anger empowers us to feel positive in our ability to change our situation and empowers us to take action.

- ❖ **Anger is a bargaining tool**. It flares when someone or something has challenged our personal value or welfare and helps us to bargain to our advantage.

- ❖ **Anger fosters cooperation.** Justifiable anger with an appropriate level of expression tells others we are entitled to the expectation of cooperation and compromise.

- ❖ **Anger gives us insight into our deeper issues.** Anger can present as a covering layer for the fear of being hurt, alone, rejected, abandoned, or unloved. This is why it is so important to find the true source of the anger and address the underlying issue. By addressing the root cause, we find solutions.

- ❖ **Anger leads to self-improvement.** When anger shows us our shortcomings, we can choose to improve, thereby improving our lives and relationships.

- ❖ **Anger promotes a sense of self-worth**. Allowing ourselves to acknowledge our anger tells us we have the intrinsic value for equitable treatment. A stronger sense of self-worth increases our emotional intelligence and wisdom, helping us to become more adaptive and resilient to the challenges we face.

Managing Anger

The core of healthy anger management is effective communication, but that doesn't come easily for everyone. It definitely did not come easy for me as my initial reaction was to repress anything I felt. My other knee jerk reaction to expressing my anger was to say something entirely stupid to the wrong person. Then, I would end up having to apologize for getting angry as well as for whatever stupid thing I said.

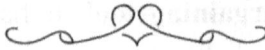

Many years ago, I was told a story that perfectly illustrates how anger builds up and comes out wrong. A young man had a flat on his car on a lonely street with just a few houses (before the days of cell phones, apparently). Since he didn't have a jack, he needed to borrow one. He went up to a house and knocked. When the resident answered, he asked them if he could borrow a jack to fix his flat. The resident slammed the door in his face.

The same thing happened at the next few houses the young man approached. Discouraged but without any other options, he went up to the last house but when the door opened, he shouted, "You can keep your damned jack!"

This is so me.

The overwhelming flood of emotions that kick in immediately in response to an injustice can make you feel powerless, defenseless, and vulnerable to whatever is thrown at you. Anger is an instinctive reactive process but handling the situation happens only after calming the lizard brain enough so the rational brain can do the communicating.

Here are some things you can do to help gather yourself to react to a situation without being reactive.

Think before you react. If you are a person who needs a minute to process what was said or done to you, that's okay. Not everyone can fire off an intelligent, well-placed comeback; and if that doesn't describe you, know it is okay to take a minute and gather your thoughts before you react or say anything. In the moment, it feels like you have to immediately defend yourself but that isn't true.

Try to calm yourself before you react. Here is where taking a few deep breaths can help. Stress causes us to breathe quickly and shallowly. When we take a few deep breaths, we shift out of our survival brain reactions into our thinking brains as tension is released. Getting away from the situation can help. Walking away, getting some alone time, or doing a mini mental escape are all effective techniques to help you reduce the emotions and tension in your body so you can respond deliberately.

Figure out why you are angry. Sometimes the reason you are angered is blatantly obvious but sometimes you may be reacting in response to something else, some past injustice, or even some internal, unnamed fear. Be brave enough to look at where the anger is coming from.

Let go of that which you cannot control. The root of the first few phases of grief, denial, anger, and bargaining are all born of an effort to control what is happening to us. Control is a survival mechanism. We believe we have to control certain aspects of ourselves and our environment to ensure our survival. The deep need to try to control what we can does not mean we are control freaks. We just need to learn when to let go. Letting go of control is terrifying when faced with a breast cancer diagnosis. We may need to fight for control of some aspect of what is happening and that is perfectly okay. Loss of control feels like powerlessness and letting go of control may feel like giving up. Being forced to surrender triggers fears and manifests in anger over things that, at any other time, may not bother us at all.

Think of the best way to handle the triggering situation before you react. Trying all the suggestions listed above is important because they stop you from coming from the perspective of the reactive lizard brain. The idea is that getting past the reactive phase will ensure you are speaking using your rational thinking brain. Sometimes saying something to set a person straight or prevent them from doing whatever is bothering you is necessary.

Sometimes you will be wasting time and energy they do not deserve. You can't educate trolls, fix stupid, or change those who refuse to do so. Be cautiously selective about whom you express your anger to. In an abusive situation, expressing your anger can be dangerous. Children do not necessarily understand where your anger comes from and tend to believe they are at fault. Tenuous relationships can be damaged by expressing anger creating lasting problems. Sometimes the best action is no reaction at all. You have to get your rational brain online to find the best solution to the situation.

Express yourself. This is the time you get to open your mouth. Hopefully you have created a masterpiece comeback, but if not, know you are in good company. Keeping your tone of voice even and measured is helpful. Using non-confrontational I-statements are crucial to clear communication and conflict resolution. "I'm upset because you said/did that." "I don't appreciate your saying that." "I feel hurt when you say/do things like that." Try to avoid criticism or placing blame. You are entitled to say what you feel and do not have to justify your feelings to anyone else. Be assertive, not aggressive.

Recognize that most people do not handle correction well, and that is not your problem. The greater number of people struggle with correction or criticism and will immediately defend themselves, which opens the door to more injustices and anger. They may rationalize why they said what they did or make you be the bad guy in some way—anything to take the responsibility of their words and actions off themselves. Some people have an overwhelming need to be right and will fight for their point of view to the death. Some will get defensive or passive aggressive. They may react in anger or get emotional, getting their feelings hurt from your confronting them. You are not responsible for their coping mechanisms and reactions as long as you are coming from that calm, rational brain line of communication.

Search for ways to defuse the underlying tension of anger that is directed toward things you cannot control, like breast cancer. Find little ways to control your environment. If you can't control having to get chemotherapy, pack a bag of your favorite comfort items to have with you. You can't control the fact that you got breast cancer, but you can control your diet, smoking, and choosing to take care of yourself. Or not. Choosing to continue with unhealthy lifestyle measures is a way of controlling your environment too. Those choices may bite in the long run, but you are still in control.

Let off some steam. Sometimes your emotions don't have a physical target like when you are angry at cancer, God, or health care systems. Energy can be released in a healthy way by destroying something that has little consequences, buying you time by reducing your reactivity. For example, you can purchase cheap dishes at a flea market and go somewhere safe to smash them to bits. Or you can buy some crummy stuffed animals at a secondhand store and lock yourself in your garage with a pair of scissors or a knife and whack away until stuffing is floating about your ears like snow. You can even get Dammit Dolls on Amazon. (I read some reviews where people didn't like the fact that they couldn't pick the fabric pattern but would receive a random choice. Good thing they had the Dammit Doll in hand to take out their frustrations about fabric options upon.)

Try exercise if you can. Not all anger is destructive and can elicit some powerful creative expression. The endorphins released with exercise will help defuse your anger.

Engage in creative outlets. Writing, journaling, painting, or any expression of what you are feeling can help transfer the emotion from your body to outside of yourself. It is a myth that anger is solely a destructive emotion.

Release the blame. First of all, forgive yourself for getting angry. Anger is simply your lizard brain functioning well. Handling anger inappropriately is something you can change, too. Then, release the grudge against others. Holding a list in your heart of those who have wronged you hurts only you. With your rational brain online, you may be able to see what drove the person to do or say what they did and empathize. Forgiveness is a powerful tool. Holding the negativity of anger and resentment crowds out positive feelings leaving you bitter and unhappy. Forgiveness does not mean the injustice was right or that you deserved what has happened. It just means you can remember the injustice and how it made you feel but you no longer feel the anger or resentment when you have to interact with the person in the future. When your anger is direct-ed at an unseen force such as cancer, the resolve to find good in what comes out of the process is a way of taking your power back.

Know when you need help. Everyone has trouble controlling anger at times. If anger is causing you a lot of distress, seems out of control, or you are doing or saying things that are causing harm, seek help from a professional. There's no shame in needing help.

I've gone so far in-depth about anger for a reason. Even though the momentary flash of anger from someone's insensitive remark or lack of support when you need it the most can be so small it seems inconsequential, unresolved anger is too dangerous to fluff over. During cancer treatment, surgery, and recovery, energy levels can be so staggeringly low that injustice doesn't seem worth the energy to get upset. Momentary irritation or anger is easy enough to repress; however, unresolved anger still leaves its mark within you.

Technically, the anger represented in this phase of the grieving process is more like the instinctive fight reaction of lizard brain. Think of the startled snapping dog. Trouble happens when there is already a long history of repressing anger where anger and self-judgment get blown out of proportion as it did for me.

Let's Make a Deal: Bargaining

May your choices reflect your hopes,
not your fears.

Nelson Mandela

In this phase, since we were unable to think or figure our way out of this mess, we then go into high gear trying to imagine a way to soften the blow. *Maybe if I do everything the doctor says, I will beat this. Maybe if I take these supplements, eat these mushrooms, or do these advanced energy healings, I won't have cancer anymore. Maybe if I find the right doctor, treatment, therapy, energy healer, shaman I will be healed. People have miracle healings all the time, why not me?*

I don't want to crush anyone's process here. Maybe you will be the one for a miracle healing. Give yourself the space to give whatever energy you need to give for the hope and belief this can happen. Give yourself permission to do whatever you need to do to achieve the outcome you are hoping for. Be warned though, chemo and many allopathic medical routes for the treatment of breast cancer advise against the use of certain supplements. If you choose this route of dual treatment, please check with your oncologist or other physician for recommendations. The modalities need to work *together*. Hiding what you are taking or doing from your medical team can get dangerous.

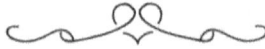

Still reeling from the shock of my diagnosis, I wandered into a health food store hoping to find some good vitamins or herbs to support me through surgery and chemo. The proprietor, who was an acquaintance of mine, was taken aback by my diagnosis. When I told her about my upcoming mastectomy, she adamantly told me that cancer treatment is barbaric and I should cancel all my appointments, take mushroom supplements, and wait to see if I died. Well, she didn't exactly say that last part but that was the implication.

She went on to say the mushrooms were really expensive, but she would help me and might even use my case as a study to prove that cancer can be cured by them. So now I'm supposed to decide whether I need to cut off my breast and go through chemo in order to live or stop all treatment, take mushroom pills, and see if I die? Or is it the other way around? And here I thought my big decision of the day was which brand of vitamins to buy.

Bargaining is the natural next step our thinking brains have to take in order to figure how to deal with our aggressor, cancer, which hasn't gone away but hasn't eaten us like the lion our instinctive bodies thought was going to happen. Our lizard brains stop pumping out fight or flight hormones and our parasympathetic nervous system starts taking over, allowing our thinking, rational brains to work. The possibilities to mitigate our situations are endless. Bargaining is what happens when we hope, pray, or wish in an exchange that an outcome will be different. Usually, this means a behavioral change or believing if we make the "right" decision the outcome will be near perfect. We can't predict the best outcome, but this is our attempt to do the best we can.

Bargaining is another way our brains can try to hold reality at bay for a while. It softens and delays the truth from settling in with all its finality creates fear and anxiety about what can happen. It can also go in a couple of different directions. One way is where our minds start hammering out thoughts of *What if?* and *If only* which serve to torment us further. *If only I had done this or not done that, this wouldn't have happened.* You may plead with God that this all be a mistake and offer to be a better person or do acts of kindness in order to receive a miracle healing. Or you may beat yourself up for all your wrong life choices and feel that cancer is your punishment for making those mistakes.

The other way bargaining shows up is thinking that if you make the right decision, it will be like it never happened or the outcome won't be as bad as your screaming lizard brain is telling you it will be. When you get diagnosed with breast cancer, decisions are flung at you fast and furiously. It is hard to take a breath, much less decide your future, when you're faced with so many high-stakes decisions.

Right after diagnosis is when you need your lizard brain pacified and your rational brain to be functional. There are countless decisions you will be asked to make: What kind of treatment approach do you want? Which cancer facility, team of medical professionals, should it be lumpectomy versus mastectomy, in the case of mastectomy do you choose one or both breasts? If you go with mastectomies, do you choose reconstruction? And, if yes to reconstruction, what type? Unfortunately, I found some people may not be given all the reconstruction options as they may not be available in certain areas. Nor may the option of having an aesthetic flat closure be mentioned. There was a collective attitude of "But of course, you want reconstruction…"

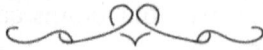

I didn't get many choices. My surgeon said my breast needed to come off because of the type and aggressiveness of my tumor. Still in shock/denial phase, those words made no sense to me. She showed me post-reconstruction photos of a woman who had bilateral nipple-sparing mastectomies. They looked better than what I was sporting at the moment, which gave me hope. However, I noticed that those photos were of a person with bilateral mastectomies. How about unilateral mastectomy photos? She didn't have any but explained that I could talk about that with the plastic surgeon.

Thank God my sweetie was there. He is the calm in my emotional storm and the logic in my irrational mind. I don't know if I could have found the door to leave without him. We both mumbled our goodbyes and left to make the same-day appointment with the plastic surgeon.

Things didn't go so great there. There was a language barrier to some extent, but he seemed kind and attentive enough. I just couldn't understand what he was telling us the reconstruction would look like. We were shown a torso-only photo of an apparently elderly woman with huge, pendulous breasts. It looked like a before surgery shot because there was no scarring and as a nurse, I've seen lots of breasts. Those hadn't seen a scalpel. I'm wondering why on earth was he showing us someone's before surgery photos? And he was comparing me to this person? Was he telling me that's what I looked like? I have a mirror at home, thank you very much. Besides, admittedly yes, they have traveled south but I couldn't tuck them in my panties yet so what was he saying? Was he saying that was what I would look like? Dear Lord, please don't give me the bosom of an eighty-year-old lady until I get there. It scared the daylights out of me.

It sounded like this doctor was telling me I was going to get a huge implant on the left and let it swing like a bowling ball on my front so it would hang level with my remaining breast. He went on to suggest a smaller implant on the right (healthy breast) to get them to match better. My lizard brain was screaming so loudly that I couldn't think. I asked about other types of reconstruction, but he wouldn't talk about them because they were not available to me unless I went out of state. Then, he waited for me to answer only I couldn't remember the question. My husband helped by telling the doctor he thought I was scared by the photos he showed me. I could only nod because my voice left me. I walked out of there wondering if I was going to feel and look like a freak afterward. No wonder I had nightmares.

Looking back, I don't believe I ever asked my husband what he thought I should do as far as reconstruction. He never tried to influence me in any direction, but I could always feel his support for whatever I chose. Desperately trying to choose the "right" thing, my brain became a storm of all the horrific outcomes for any of my choices. We had twenty-nine years of marriage together, and I didn't believe he was the type to walk out on me, but I worried he wouldn't want me sexually anymore. I feared the revulsion I might see in his eyes.

The trouble is that all the questions come at a time when you are not adequately equipped to make the best decisions for yourself. Even though the initial shock begins to fade, the fears and possibilities are coming at you so fast and with an urgency that you feel you can't take the time to consider what is the best decision for you.

Right after a cancer diagnosis is also the time that the decisions can be crucial, even though we are still actively grieving having gotten cancer in the first place. If we have not allowed ourselves time and grace to fully process the shock, denial, and initial anger of the diagnosis, we will still be flooded with all those fight or flight hormones. Our rational brains cannot make themselves be heard until our reactiveness and fears are calmed down to some extent. It would be great if someone just diagnosed with breast cancer had time to rest before having to make life-altering decisions but that doesn't typically happen.

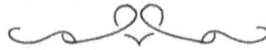

From the day I was diagnosed to the day I had my mastectomy, which was the first step to getting free of cancer, there were fifty-one days of sheer mental hell. I was supposed to patiently wait for the surgery room and two surgeons' operating schedules to magically align. In the meantime, I felt like I had a bomb in my breast that could explode at any second, sending cancer throughout my body. It wasn't like I had a choice, so I waited. Just me and my industrial-strength imagination that can zero in on all things negative like a heat-seeking missile.

I paced the floors at 2 a.m. trying not to wake my husband but unable to stop the madness of terror chattering in my head that kept me from sleep. What precious little sleep I got was riddled with nightmares. Am I going to be mutilated? What will my reconstructed breast look like? What if I make the wrong decision? What if I die in surgery? What if it metastasizes and I die of breast cancer? What should I do? Am I doing the right thing? I asked my surgeon why there was such a wait to get to surgery and she tried to reassure me that my case wasn't urgent. Well, maybe my cancer wasn't urgent but my level of anxiety was.

Cancer is not an urgent condition, says anyone who isn't waiting for an opening in a surgery schedule.

My best advice around this waiting period right after diagnosis is don't do it the way I did. Anything but that will be an improvement. Speak up to your doctors, ask for help. If you need to talk to a professional counselor, ask for it. If you can't sleep, talk to your doctor. Ask for what you need and keep asking. This doesn't have to be a hellish time for you.

Many insurances do not provide counseling without considerable copays. That means that people unable to afford the copays do not have the option to seek help. Nor are professional counselors available in all areas. As a part of my mission, I hope to see that all people diagnosed with breast cancer have immediate access to mental and emotional support. I want to raise awareness that mental and emotional health are vital to good physical health outcomes and crucial to ongoing quality of life. Support needs to be a part of the treatment plan from the start, giving as much attention and respect to a person's emotional well-being as their physical health. Although such support groups do exist in some cancer centers, I hope to see it universalized and available to all.

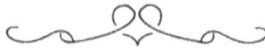

My treatment was at UAMS, a teaching hospital in Little Rock over an hour drive from home. While I wandered around waiting to be called back for appointments, I looked for anything offered for cancer patients. I saw a class offered called Look Good/Feel Better which would be nice, but I couldn't see wrapping a two-and-a-

half-hour drive to come learn how to do makeup. My oncologist suggested a group that met weekly at the hospital to talk and offer advice and support to each other. I would be able to learn how to manage details like where to get wigs and such. Since the group didn't meet on my chemo days when I was in the city, I couldn't make it, and I sure didn't have the energy to make another commute.

I already had a wig anyway.

Having cancer is stressful enough but there are many changes and decisions to be made outside of treatment. You may have to balance your job or work around your treatment schedule, energy levels, and potential brain fog that affects your performance. Childcare, carpooling, after school events, cooking, cleaning, and all the bazillion chores we do as parents still have to be done. The desire to keep children's lives unaffected by what you are going through is strong, so strong that you put your needs last and potentially harm yourself.

Stress builds creating anxiety, which in turn, causes burnout. I've listed a few suggestions for releasing stress. I can't vouch for them personally since I blundered through this time doing everything wrong, but I do them now. They do work.

Accept yourself for how you feel. Exercise a little self-compassion by understanding that this is a time you are not able to control the outcome. All you can control is how you handle this experience. That starts with acknowledging and accepting what is right now without judgment.

Try grounding exercises. When we are tense or anxious, we pull our energy up into our torso. Our hearts beat faster, our throats can feel constricted, or our stomachs feel upset. Take a moment and feel the pressure of your feet against the floor or your buttocks against the chair you are sitting in. Focus on the sensation of support from your surroundings. Doing so tells your body you are safe at this moment and may calm the tightness in your chest.

Explore mindfulness. We operate on autopilot way too often. Try focusing or paying close attention to what you are doing while noticing from a place of curiosity, the feelings and sensations that come. Walking is an example. Notice details of what you see and hear, the sun on your face, or the sound of your heels striking the ground. Eating is another. How often do we sit down to eat and then notice the food is all gone but have no memory of how or where it went, much less what it tasted like after the first few bites? Mindfulness pulls us away from the fears of the future to the safety of the present.

Find a healthy distraction. Try music, watching movies or TV, reading, or your favorite creative outlet. Activate your senses by taking luxurious baths, enjoying your favorite essential oils in a diffuser, dancing, or intense exercise. Sneak in some mindfulness by returning to your focus when your thoughts wander.

Try a mantra or words of encouragement. Come up with a mantra you can repeat anytime you need encouragement. Positive affirmations are powerful in flipping negative thought patterns into positive ones. Good examples are: "I'm strong and I can get through this." "I'm in charge of how I feel, and I choose to feel calm and relaxed." "I'm worthy, deserving, and enough." If your mind starts screaming that you are lying to yourself, modify the mantra to something you can believe such as "I'm learning to be stronger" or "I know that I am enough." The Serenity Prayer works for some. Psalm 23 was my personal favorite. In my head, it was the King James Version. The ancient language felt comforting.

Encourage a sense of appreciation or gratitude. It is incredibly easy to forget what is good in our lives when things go wrong. I'm not talking about adding more "should" talk in our lives like "We should be more grateful" because it can always be worse. It can. But negating what is happening to you or how you feel does not create gratitude. It is another way of beating yourself up for not being or feeling differently. Instead, search around you for something you like which you can feel, see, smell, or have and give a moment of thanks that it is there, and you have the ability to enjoy it.

Keep engaged in your life. It's natural to want to go into hiding or put your life on hold while you are worried, scared, or anxious but the resulting isolation feeds into fear. It makes you feel more anxious and alone. Keep doing what you normally enjoy doing and with someone you enjoy being around. Regardless of how things turn out for you in the future, you won't regret the good you experience in the meantime.

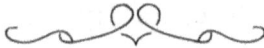

My encounter with the health food store proprietor left me reeling with more fears about making the right decisions for me. I am a believer in alternative and allopathic medicine. I have studied Traditional Chinese Medicine, herbal therapies, and some energy practices. I'm still an advanced practice nurse with a long and rich medical background. It's like having a foot in two vastly different worlds. So which way do I go? Holistic therapies including a blend of methodologies such as acupuncture, herbal therapy, yoga, meditation, or biofeedback with chemo-therapy and radiation wasn't as mainstream then as they are now.

Finally, after much self-induced mental torture, I decided to imagine I was making a decision. First, I tried the option of alternative mushroom supplements and canceling all future doctor appointments. I visualized myself walking a path and pictured holding the capsules in my hand, lifting them to my mouth to swallow. I envisioned myself using my phone to call and cancel my upcoming doctor appointments. I thought about the healthy meals and practices I would adopt. The longer I practiced this visualization, I started noticing how anxious I was getting. Something about this path was making me nervous. It was time to try the other path.

My scheduled appointment with my breast surgeon was the next day, which I decided to keep. I showed up for the appointment with the awareness that I was going to see how doing as she suggested made me feel. I wasn't committing to anything by going. Sitting naked from the waist up in my little cloth wrap nervously anticipating her arrival, my husband and I waited. She strode into the clinic room, sat down, and turned to me. In that instant, a soft, warm, buttery sense of peace descended over me. It was so compelling that I could not deny I was in the right place with the right surgeon. No matter what happened afterward, I knew I was making the right decision for me.

Believing in the ability to make the best decisions for yourself will come easy for some and not for others. I was one of the latter group. I canvased many people's opinions, researched, drew upon my medical background, sought multiple opinions from the medical community of which I was a member, meditated for all the good that did, and prayed, no, beseeched God to help me. When my prayers seemingly went unanswered, I felt I was somehow flawed and unlovable by God. My rational mind knew better but my heart didn't.

Trying to make the best decisions for yourself is hard enough but when you take in everyone's opinion, things get really rocky. It is easy to get lost in not trusting yourself to make the best decisions for yourself because the stakes are too high. I follow a few Facebook support groups and see many women posting questions about what everyone else chose, how it turned out for them, or simply asked the group what they should do. The answers are as varied as snowflakes. Everyone has an opinion, most feel their opinion is the absolute truth, but you can be assured there won't be a definite right answer for you. If you find yourself asking the opinion of perfect strangers, you aren't the only one to do so.

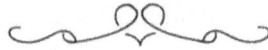

⁂

I practically polled everyone I saw as to what I should choose about my mastectomy and reconstruction. I got a lot of strange looks. Anyway, my breast surgeon told me my cancer was in my left, and my right breast was healthy, therefore a bilateral mastectomy was not necessary. Her words rearranged themselves in my head to say I could only have the left removed and reconstructed. I didn't question it.

I also got the surgery date screwed up. Those words playing Scrabble in my head made me think my surgery date was set so I contacted my boss like a good little employee and scheduled time off. I worked for the State of Arkansas in women's health clinics. My work week found me in five different county health clinics. Taking off work meant a huge undertaking of rearranging already tight nurse practitioners' schedules, canceling or rescheduling clients' appointments, and getting the clients their extra birth control so they could make it until they could be seen. My boss got my clients covered just before I found out that I got the dates wrong, and it was really two weeks later. I hesitantly told my supervisor I had misunderstood, and could she please let me have all my clients back for two more weeks and then go through her massive shuffling system again. To her credit, I only heard her give a deep shaky breath before saying okay.

Two weeks flew by pretty fast, and my mind was made up. I was going to have a unilateral mastectomy with reconstruction. To start the reconstruction, an expander was to be placed where the implant would fit. It would be gradually filled with small amounts of saline over a period of weeks. The purpose of the expander was to give my skin and chest wall muscle time to stretch and adjust to the size of the upcoming implant. It was going to be okay, and I started to relax. Finally, I was doing something proactive to get through having breast cancer.

The time came for me to sign the consent form, so I showed up for my appointment feeling confident in my decision.

Before any kind of surgery, a health care professional has to discuss with you the exact surgery planned, tell you the risks, and field any questions you have. I was sitting in a cramped little closet-sized exam room where a young doctor-in-training was giving me this information and wanting me to sign the consent form for my upcoming surgery in a teaching medical center. He read the part about having a unilateral mastectomy and got a startled look on his face. He asked me why I wasn't having bilateral surgery. I answered honestly that I thought I couldn't because I only had cancer on one side. Here is undeniable proof that all that you know can fly out the window when you are staring down the barrel of a gun because I, nurse practitioner extraordinaire, should have known better. Of course, I could have chosen a bilateral if that was what I wanted.

He got my surgeon to come in and talk to me about having a bilateral. She said I would be fine no matter which decision I made. It was totally up to me.

Well, isn't that just GREAT. I had just spent the last eight weeks agonizing over the impending loss of one breast and now I had to make a snap decision whether to whack them both. The pro is there would be no future worries about cancer and symmetry of my reconstructed breasts. Trust me, I had enough nightmares about having one breast perched under my collar bone and the other tucked into my waistband. But the con would be cutting off a healthy breast with real live sensations unlike the numb implant I expected.

Another kink in the system was that if I chose a bilateral mastectomy instead of my unilateral, the time slot for my surgery room was only enough time to do one breast. That meant I would have to cancel surgery and be rescheduled for a later date. For nearly two months, I had been driving myself insane in fear and now here was my chance to extend it even longer until another surgery room with both surgeons' schedules magically aligned... again.

Fears warred with common sense until a tornado of indecision obliterated any rational thought. I looked to my husband in desperation and saw clearly the unspoken message in his eyes. No way could he make this decision for me. I looked at the wannabe-doctor and saw him mentally drumming his fingers in impatience. Dr. Wannabe finally spoke up and said, "You seem to me to be a person who can't make up her mind very easily."

Anyone with two functional brain cells would know that this was NOT what you say to someone in this situation. He needed to get an attitude adjustment big time. If it were not my breasts but his balls on the chopping block, I bet he would do some stuttering, too. You would also think that I, with my extensive health care experience and understanding of therapeutic communication, would be the one to enlighten him. What did I do? I apologized for taking so long.

I ended up going for the unilateral with reconstruction initially. Opting to keep my healthy boob seemed like a good call. (I did not know I would be facing a mastectomy of the right breast in just one year.) I signed the consent, and it was full speed ahead for my set surgery date. Besides, no way in hell was I calling my supervisor and telling her she had to rearrange the clinic schedules for a third time.

There is also a danger of putting too much energy into trying to think your way through what is to come or how things will turn out. When it doesn't go well, it is easy to think that it is because you did something wrong or that good outcomes are for everyone but you. And nothing could be further from the truth.

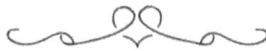

Facebook wasn't on my radar the year I got breast cancer, but in late 2012, I got with the times and created my profile. I rarely posted but kept up with others' posts even if it was just pictures of what they were about to eat. Then Facebook ads started rolling in my newsfeed. It took a while, but I noticed that Facebook knows everything about its users. I had joined a couple of BC groups to see what they were like. Ten minutes later, my feed was inundated with ads for specialty bras and cancer treatment options.

The hardest ads to see were the ones where someone cured their incurable cancer with dietary changes, supplements, meditation, affirmations, or a combination of each. It made me think that maybe I was wrong to go through all

I did with my mastectomy, reconstruction, and chemo-therapy. My anxiety would shoot up as I scrambled to shut my phone down so I wouldn't have to see them. Why couldn't I have been one of the magically healed? Did that mean I was not as good, special, worthy, or important enough to get a miracle? What if the cure for breast cancer comes the day after I go through all my hellish treatments?

It's not like I don't believe in miracles. It just made me wonder why it didn't happen for me. Maybe if I had only known and bought their course I would have been cured. Maybe if I had done anything else, I would have gotten the cure and kept my breasts, too. Maybe I could spend the rest of my life wishing I had done something else. Maybe I could just continue to beat myself up for making the decisions I had made.

It took me forever to decide what was best for me and now there I was, second guessing every decision I made. I couldn't go back and change what I'd done. I could only go forward and make the best of each day. Beating myself up for what I coulda shoulda woulda done wasn't doing it for me anymore.

Meanwhile, I'd lost a few pounds and could use some new underwear. I wondered what size to order. I bet Facebook knows.

———————

The best answer for you will come *from* you, not some outside source. No one will be able to decide what the best treatment option is for you unless you feel good about it. It is really easy to hop up on the conveyor belt of the medical system and hand over all your power and responsibility in the process. Deciding to let someone else make all your decisions is possibly the only wrong decision a person can make. It may be nice to be able to blame someone else if the outcome turns out bad, but the goal is to know you made the best decision for yourself so there is no need to second guess your decisions no matter what the outcome.

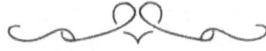

Sometimes in an effort to connect with others who spoke my language of breast cancer, I would go shop at a post-mastectomy supply and apparel shop in my town. I would wander the racks and talk with the owners and other customers, discussing everything from the most comfortable bras to our experiences feeling included in a special band of people who had gone through similar challenges.

One busy day, the shop was filled with shoppers browsing the racks along with me. A woman, maybe about ten years younger than I approached me and asked if I had gotten reconstruction. She was really cute and slim wearing an open jean jacket, darling little top, and chunky necklace all of which made me instantly jealous, but I smiled and told her yes, I had. She got a strange look on her face and said she hadn't. She said she thought it more important that she be there for her children. She instantly pivoted around and strode out of the shop.

Watching her retreating back, my brain went into self-doubt overload. Was my reconstruction a selfish, vain move? Would it have been more noble to not have gotten reconstruction? I was prepared for outsiders to not under-stand what I'd been through, but to get this from one of my own hit hard.

Then, the cobwebs that inhabited my brain started to clear. She, as I, made the best decision she could with what resources she had at the time. She must have been having some doubt as to the wisdom of her choices since then, so she needed to reassure herself that she did the right thing. Her statement wasn't a judgment that her decision was better than mine even though it sure felt that way.

My experiences are in no way a judgment of anyone else's. They are simply mine. There is no right or wrong way, just the best way available for you and me in the moment. How others manage their experiences is no reflection on how to get through breast cancer. You do you and I do me. If we can support each other because we have special insight into the trauma of breast cancer, all the better.

It took me a while to tame the beast called my self-judgment and see that what she said was not personal at all. She was probably hurting for some reason I wasn't aware of. As for me, I truly regret that she didn't hang around for us to talk a bit. I really wanted to know where she got her jean jacket.

————————

For those who find themselves in this phase needing to make tough decisions and feeling overwhelmed, self-trust is key. I asked God for neon-flashing billboards that spelled out what I should do but they never appeared, and they probably won't for you either. What happened was that I had to trust myself to make the best decision with the information I had at the time and let the rest go. Then when things didn't go as planned, I had the confidence to make the best of whatever came. No longer did I take the outcome personally but appreciated the good and the lessons of the bad. When you are able to make your decisions with confidence, you will realize that none of your decisions are technically wrong.

People have a variety of ways they make decisions. Some people use a visceral gut feeling to clue them toward the direction that is best for them. Inner knowledge or a sensation of knowing but not knowing how you know it can help as guidance. Intuition can show in many different ways if we would only pay attention. Observing for clues or signs (not necessarily the billboard type I asked God for) that appear in our outer environment to confirm or induce caution for a potential decision is good. Look inside of yourself for that inner sense of peace, awareness, or quiet "click" that tells you it is the right choice.

Learning and researching all you can about your options is good for making informed decisions but to try to figure out or predict the future based on your thoughts while ignoring your inner guidance spells danger. To listen and act upon your inner voice or wisdom will take faith but faith grows with action. A word of caution here: Having a strong emotional attachment to the decision will cause you to confuse or override your inner nudge. That inner voice is quiet and easily drowned out.

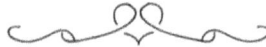

I felt confident a mastectomy and future chemo was the way to go for me. However, I got a sick feeling about the reconstruction part. All I was told about reconstruction was how great it was. How it would be like no one could ever tell I had breast cancer. Still, I felt like I was having a panic attack every time I thought about it. I tried to research reconstruction options, but they were limited to two: an expander placed the day of the mastectomy which was filled gradually over a period of weeks or an implant placed the same day as surgery. The second one was discouraged as the end result may not be as aesthetically pleasing.

Convinced it was just fears of how I would look, I gave up worrying about it and figured the plastic surgeon knew what was best. I went for Option A.

What I didn't know was that it hurt like hell. The tissue and skin of my breast didn't heal well, and the initial implant failed. I eventually had another mastectomy (my remaining breast) and reconstruction of both breasts so the process was really strung out, but I didn't know that it would take six surgeries total including repairs before I had the seventh and final surgery—explants to flat.

The skin over my left implant had such poor blood supply it looked purple and dead. Nobody told me I wouldn't be able to lie on my stomach at all and lying on my side was too painful. In fact, any touch was too painful. Forget having my husband touch them. They were incredibly numb, itchy, and painful all at the same time. Wearing a bra was out of the question. My shoulders became so inflamed that I lost all my range of motion. I couldn't fold a sheet and hanging up clothes in the closet was excruciating. I had T-rex arms glued to my sides. Even reaching to clean myself on the toilet was intensely painful and brought tears to my eyes.

Also, I wasn't prepared for how they would look. I hoped for a nice breast shape and what I got was horrific caricatures. My Frankenboobs. They were misshapen and stuck to my pectoral muscles which meant that every movement of my arms caused them to shoot up to my armpits. You just can't hide that level of ugly. I couldn't wear a bra and my clothes clung to them, so I hunched over to hide them, which increased my shoulder and back pain.

I had totally ignored that inner voice urging for no reconstruction. I wasn't ready to give up breasts and dreamed they would be what I was told they could be. My fear during the first surgery was of being disfigured with no breast on the left and my natural breast remaining on the right. I hang pictures with a laser level. Symmetry is huge in my eyes. So huge, in fact, that I fought my inner voice that my reconstruction was not right for me so hard that I obliterated it.

Writing about my experience is especially hard because I don't want to instill more fear in people faced with decisions for reconstruction. Like I've said before, you have to follow what you believe is correct for you. There are probably reconstruction success stories out there. My story wasn't one of them. However, even though I went through reconstruction disasters to explants, what I didn't know was I would eventually feel like a total boobless badass with my slightly concave chest stuck out proudly and my arms swinging freely.

Looking back over all my early days, I cannot deny that I made the right decision for myself in electing to have the mastectomies and chemotherapy. That doesn't mean that everything came out the way I hoped it would. Nor does it mean that all of the eight billion decisions I made as a result of choosing my treatment plan would turn out all puppy cuddles and fairy dust. I have wishes and regrets. What I regretted most was giving up my power and allowing others to make decisions for me.

What I do not regret is who I became as a result of my decisions. Some decisions were easy, some were the stuff of nightmares but every one of my decisions, good or bad, were mine. They brought me fresh perspectives that I allowed to become a part of me. Even though I could not control most of what happened to me, how I chose to respond is all me. The badass me.

Here are the key points to remember when making your decisions:

- ❖ Believe that no one knows what is best for you more than you do.

- ❖ Learn all you can about your options.

- ❖ Seek professional, not anecdotal advice.

- ❖ Acknowledge that if things do not turn out the way you envision, it doesn't necessarily mean you made a mistake. Learn what you can from any experience.

- ❖ Make a pact with yourself that whatever route you choose, you will not beat yourself up in the future about it. You did the best you could at the time.

Some people will think that if they concentrate hard enough or make the right "bargain" they will get the outcome they want. However, if they focus all their energy on a certain result, they can miss ways to adapt to what is happening in the moment. Also, if there is only one acceptable outcome in their minds, any other possibility is seen as a failure. This all-or-nothing thinking is dangerous because there is no controlling the future. We can only control how we handle, process, and adapt to what is happening in the moment. Since at this stage, your body is still being flooded with stress hormones and lizard brain is still online, decisions which need to come from the analytical thinking brain are not easily made.

Friends and family as well as your medical team can also put the pressure of bargaining on you. No matter how well-intentioned their advice is, they are putting their expectations on you and that equates to pressure to conform to what they believe is right for you.

Children, especially, tend to take responsibility for everything including a mother's cancer. They can make fantastical bargains in their heads such as "if I be good, mom's cancer will go away."

When that doesn't happen, the children can internalize the failure as rejection of them. The grieving process of breast cancer is not limited to just the patient but encompasses everyone who loves and cares for them.

Any preexisting fears or judgment about cancer or the treatment can have a huge impact on how well you tolerate treatment and recovery no matter what you decide to do. For instance, if you have a latent belief that your cancer is a form of punishment for not being perfect or cancer spells certain death, healing can be much more difficult. Our minds have lots of control over how we feel, how we respond, and how we heal.

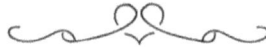

When I was back at work after chemo, I was barely functioning. I still wore scarves to cover up my new peach fuzz growing in. I still had that haggard, gray look about me but, hey, I was putting one foot in front of the other. I had a pretty light day and was looking forward to the upcoming weekend. One of my last patients for the day was a lady in her late forties who was needing a pap smear and to be set up for a mammogram. I'm grateful for these clients because generally these visits were pretty basic and uncomplicated. Or so I thought.

I started in with my routine assessment questions and things were flowing nicely, so I got started with her breast exam. She looked up at me and gently asked if I had cancer. One look at me and that answer was blatantly obvious, but this is the usual, kind way many approach the topic when they care to talk or ask about it. I have a memorized script for just this situation. These are ladies who are going for a mammogram and to see me battling cancer can be really uncomfortable. It drags the possibility of getting cancer right in their faces so I try to be sensitive to the fact that seeing me in treatment can increase worry that they, too, can get breast cancer.

I started to tell her yes but also how important it is to get your mammograms regularly, to do self-exams routinely, and that she can be comforted by the fact that early detection can greatly improve outcomes. It was a "Yes, I got breast cancer, but you can be encouraged because look how great I'm doing" kind of message. I barely got past the word yes before she was telling me I had the devil in me to have gotten cancer and that I was ignorant of the Lord to not have gotten perfect healing. My hands still busy with her breast exam, my jaw dropped in shock.

She started a tirade of scriptures proving how I was bound for hell that lasted through her entire exam. I got her to move down on the table and put her feet into the stirrups in position for her pap smear while she was still practically shouting scriptures. I tried to ask if she thought God gave doctors and the medical field the wisdom to help people and even tried to insert a few scriptures of my own. Thinking I was even a close match with her knowledge of scriptures and the willingness to regurgitate them at deafening volumes was a mistake. I shut up and completed the fastest pelvic exam in medical history. You would think that if you were flat on your back on a gyn table with me all up in your business with pointy objects, you wouldn't necessarily want to try to convince me that I'm devil possessed.

Internally, I was screaming to get out the room as fast as I could. The volume and speed of scriptures she was yelling at me was, to say the least, impressive, but I was getting really upset. One hand on the door, I hesitated. She was still shouting scriptures at me, but I slowly turned and looked at her. She finally took what must have been her first *breath in fifteen minutes and paused the onslaught. I asked her if that was how she felt, why was she here for these tests. She was momentarily speechlessness, then she said she was just making sure she was doing the right thing. Maybe in her mind, getting a normal mammogram was proof of her religious well-being. I turned and left the room.*

Leaning back against the closed exam room door, I couldn't stop shaking. Thankfully, I don't share her beliefs because if I did, I'm doomed. It took me a while to push her opinions out of my head and my heart. If I believed she was right, none of the decisions I'd made about my treatment mattered. I would have to believe that I deserved to get cancer. It would mean I didn't deserve help or to get better. Essentially, I didn't deserve to live. Imagine how well that would fit into a healing process.

The bargaining phase of the grief process can be misunderstood as a negative time where our minds fight for control of what is happening to us. If we shift that to the thought that this is where we naturally seek out all avenues of our experience in order to achieve the optimal outcome, it's possible to see the work our brains are putting in as positive and empowering. It is a choice to look at a situation and search out answers for ourselves. This is what we are designed to do, first for survival and then to maximize benefits while mitigating any damages that might occur.

By accepting this process as being normal, expected, and even helpful, we can relax into that inner feeling of peace that comes with making the best decision for ourselves. We all have an internal guidance system. We just have several different names for it. However, we have been conditioned to ignore it for the sake of others. Practicing self-trust develops our awareness and appreciation of this guidance system but it starts with self-acceptance. It starts with believing that we are the masters of our lives. We have the right to choose what we believe is best for us no matter how it impacts anyone else. We have the right and grace to get "wrong" sometimes because that is where we learn. What is sometimes misunderstood as "mistakes" are really learning opportunities about what doesn't work for us. Through our experiences, good and bad, we gain wisdom.

We are unique, unparalleled, and irreplaceable. These are our lives—our futures—on the line, and no one gets a bigger say in what happens to us than we do. Give yourself all the time and grace to come to your inner peace about what you want. That is when you will know that no matter what happens, no matter how the future unfolds, you made the best decision for yourself possible. Avoid looking for approval or basing your decisions on the advice of those who don't have to live with the consequences. Gather all the information you can and believe in yourself. Then you can move on without hesitation or wasting your precious time second-guessing your choices.

Black Cloud Days:
Depression

*When our days become dreary with low-hovering
clouds of despair, and when our nights become
darker than a thousand midnights, let us remember
that there is a creative force in this universe,
working to pull down the gigantic mountains of
evil, a power that is able to make a way out of no
way and transform dark yesterdays into bright
tomorrows.*

Martin Luther King, Jr.

Depression is one of the phases in the grieving process and one of the hardest to understand, manage, and weather. The level of judgment and the misconceptions around depression are staggering. There isn't just one type of depression and some of us who already suffer with it will get a cancer diagnosis, which makes dealing with everything in life that much more difficult. If you have a diagnosis of clinical depression, or suspect that you do, and are not being seen by a professional, dealing with that plus this phase can put you in an unsafe situation that this section is not able to adequately address. All depression is not created equally.

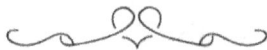

I had Maggie, my little Lord-only-knows-the-breed rescue dog for seven years when I was diagnosed with

breast cancer. From the moment I came home from my mastectomy, she tried to get close to me. She wasn't used to being away from me for any length of time. Once I was tucked into bed, she was allowed to approach where she probably got a good whiff of my drains and surgery-related stench. She cautiously walked across the bed to my side. Careful to not touch me, she sat, shaking violently with her little eyes pinched shut in terror for me. I reached out a hand to let her know I was okay. The moment I touched her, she curled up and laid down. From then on, she was glued to my side. I did not realize at the time that I would no longer feel normal unless I was with her.

It seems that getting cancer should be enough hell for anyone to go through, but it never stops there. Getting cancer uproots, challenges, and annihilates your belief systems about who you are and how you relate to God, the world, other people, and most certainly, yourself. A cancer diagnosis not only shoves fears of death in your face, but it also throws all of your carefully built stories about yourself into question.

Every arena of our lives, our self-worth, and lovability are laid bare. Because we are all unique individuals who have come from a vast variety of life circumstances, how we manage this part is also unique to each one of us. Our lives and experiences shape us and largely determine how well we adapt and roll with the punches. And cancer certainly gives one hell of a punch.

From an objective standpoint, depression is the natural development in the grieving process after denial, initial anger, and bargaining. Throughout the bargaining phase, our minds were frantically busy trying to "fix" or change what was happening to us. While this is natural and necessary, there was too much pressure to figure out what to do. Self-doubt flooded in causing us to question our ability to make the right decisions. Some decisions turned out good and maybe some didn't. There comes a point when we realize there is nothing more we can bargain to make cancer go away or soften the blow of losses we experience in health, privacy, body image, jobs, relationships, and more. If the bargaining phase of grief is where we analyze our situations, depression is when we start to feel them. Because of the massive disruption of dealing with cancer and all its "blessings," depression is the one phase that seems to be a struggle to overcome.

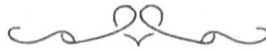

∽∽◦∾∾

I returned to work long before I was mentally or physically ready to do so. Maggie and I had become such constant companions that I was dependent on her in a way that I could not fathom. Terry, my husband, was everything I needed in a partner but still, I needed Maggie at my side. Leaving her to go to work was hard, but I could manage faking it long enough to get the job done.

When my last client had been taken care of and the last chart completed, I beelined for the door. Even though I was embarrassed to admit how dependent I had become on my little pooch, I couldn't stand to waste a second getting home to her. I stopped going shopping unless she could go in with me. Or, if she wasn't welcome and going in was unavoidable, I would leave the car locked, AC running, while I ran in. I literally barreled people over to get what I needed and back to her. When it became dangerously hot, I started grocery shopping at night. I had lots of good excuses for why I stopped leaving the house. My Amazon Prime shopping addiction soared as Maggie became my lifeline.

Going through chemo was pretty tough. I literally felt poisoned. I had no energy, everything hurt including my eyebrows. Okay, maybe not my eyebrows because I no longer had any, but you get the picture. I developed T-rex arms. You never realize what it takes for full ROM (range of motion) of the arms until you can't do it without severe pain. Forget lifting anything higher than my ribcage, hanging clothes up in the closet, or fastening a bra. Not that I needed one of those. One perk of imitation boobs from reconstruction is that they don't bounce. No bras required.

Experiencing pain twenty-four seven with post-chemo days that multiply pain exponentially really got to me. I lost interest in reading, going places, even small talk was an effort. If you're worried that chemo is that bad for everyone, the effects are really varied. You have to take into consideration your age, the "cocktail," and a gazillion other factors. In other words, there's no way of knowing how it is going to affect you. I'm just telling how it was for me.

Things that I never imagined became my new normal, like holding my breath the first pee after a chemo session. That smell was as awful as I felt. After the steroids wore off on day three, I was in bed all day unable to focus on a magazine or movie. I just lay there battling waves of pain. It's no wonder I got mentally down. Anybody would.

My one constant was Maggie at my side. She heard every moan and watched every move I made. Her steadfast loyalty every waking moment became my lighthouse in a storm. She was a blessing to me. She wasn't the only support system I had. There were family and friends checking in on me and helping any way they could. Looking back, I realize how many silent angels I had in my life, and one of those angels had paws.

Depression is a term used to describe both the sadness of going through a difficult time such as in the grieving process (situational depression) and a serious mental health condition (clinical depression) that negatively affects how you feel. They can both occur simultaneously like a layered effect, but they aren't the same. They feel differently and they need to be approached and treated differently. Clinical depression requires an entirely different treatment modality and there are particular types of depression that must be managed professionally. Not all people with preexisting clinical depression are seeking or getting the help they need so throwing in a cancer diagnosis is enough to sink the whole ship.

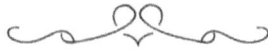

Maggie, my canine guilt monger, nagged me out of the house for a walk one day in February while I was still fresh from my chemo life. I didn't want to go. In my opinion, February is known not only for being the only month that has 11,028 days but all of said days are oppressively gray. If it weren't for her beautiful, compasssionate, melty, brown eyes that would turn into guilt-inducing laser beams drilling holes through my skull, I would have never gotten off the couch. But there I was, cold and miserable, walking behind her prancing butt. It was a really cute doggy butt. The tips of her ears flopped with each step making a smile tickle the edges of my lips. A soft, misting rain started to fall against my cheeks along with a hushed sense of peace that silenced our steps. It was magical, ours alone, and my sadness began to lift.

If we approach all types of depression alike, we either under-value this phase of situational depression, or we inappropriately manage it. Almost all information about depression relates to types of mental health conditions and gives very little credence to what we go through because of breast cancer. We are simply advised to "talk to our medical health professionals." While this is decent, appropriate advice in many cases, not everyone has the financial ability, time, or energy to do so. The lack of information that can be found makes depression seem a topic best skirted at all costs. To really understand what we feel, we need depression pulled out of the closet.

There is a lot of judgment around depression as if it is a character weakness. Sometimes depression is silently categorized as being selfish and self-absorbed, a failure to manage life in a healthy, positive way. There is a limited amount of time and patience given for a person to feel what they feel, so they'd best suck it up and get over it. Family and friends place huge pressure on you to stay positive. They generally do not always know what to say to make things better and are afraid for you to be depressed so they tend to encourage you to stay strong and only focus on the bright days. This encouragement is important at times but can put pressure on you to deny what you feel or just keep it to yourself.

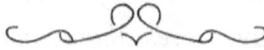

So many people came up to me with bright smiles and told me to stay strong and positive, to keep fighting. That was so easy for them to say. I was tired of needing to be strong and wanted it all to stop long enough for me to get a breath.

Loved ones initially rally around with support, and the other cancer patients you meet are inspirational. However, there come dark days that drag you down no matter how blessed you are. All the good intentions to coax you out of depression before you are ready put incredible pressure on you to at least fake it so they will either feel better or leave you alone.

Sometimes, the constant urging to stay positive and strong is the last thing you want to hear. There will be times that the encouragement feels supportive and other times that you need to know it is okay to be scared. It's okay to be sad. You don't have to keep a smile pasted to your face when all you really need is time alone or a time to be held, a time to be seen and accepted for who you are.

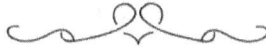

About halfway through my chemotherapy treatments, I was feeling emotionally as gray as the color of my skin. I was sitting in the exam room with my husband and my oncologist, Dr. Issam Makhoul, as new orders were written for that day's chemotherapy cocktail. Perhaps because I was so weak and listless, Dr. Makhoul was extra gentle and tender with his questions about how I was doing. I gave the expected answers and he turned to the computer to type in the orders. He glanced back at me, his eyes full of compassion, and quietly asked if there was anything I needed. I answered with a sigh and a resounding yes, because despite going through all this hell, I wasn't going to get the one thing I asked for.

He whipped around from the computer and pushed closer on his wheeled stool. Expectantly, he asked what that might be. I took a deep breath and told him I wanted a bionic boob. I would be happy with a rocket launcher or a flame thrower imitating Arnold Schwarzenegger in True Lies as I directed an imaginary flame sweeping in front of me. This is about the time I saw the blank look of utter disbelief for what he was hearing in Dr. Makhoul's eyes. His jaw dropped, and I started to get worried. My spiel wobbled a bit, not knowing if I should continue. English was not Dr. Makhoul's first language, and I had no idea how my odd humor translated across cultural divides so any sensible person would have just shut up and smiled. That is so not me.

Plowing ahead, I told him I wanted weapons of mass destruction. Or, at the very least, I should get a poison dart gun to use when someone irritated me; I could just press a button on my boob and take them out. I could feign surprise and gasp out loud, totally getting away with it. But, no, I'm getting a water balloon, a squirt gun at best. As I got more into my tale, I began to see the realization dawn in Dr. Makhoul's eyes as he started to smile, then broke into laughter. Soon we were all laughing, and I didn't feel so gray anymore. This was the first time I thought I was going to make it through this hell. I just might survive.

Situational depression is sneaky. Not many people wake up one day and realize they are feeling depressed about their lives. It can be insidious, like a tiny voice that reminds you of what all you have lost, can no longer do, no longer have the energy for, and how you are letting down everyone around you. And let's not forget that the house still needs to be cleaned and laundry done.

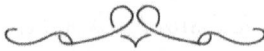

Maggie was in training as an emotional support animal but I felt like a fraud putting her vest on. The day of her final test, I was late getting off work, which made me late getting her to the testing site. I was nervous and she felt it. She did great until the last test. She was to sit quietly for five minutes while I walked away. She failed. In truth, I failed her. I couldn't hold it together long enough for her to be okay with me walking away.

I don't know if she would have gotten the certification if I would have felt differently. Having an ESA was to admit I was a person who needed emotional support. That wasn't who I wanted to be. I felt pathetic. Look at me, the professional nurse practitioner who went into panic when her little doggie wasn't nearby.

I stopped seeing friends and family if she couldn't come. My life became dominated by my need to be with her. I kept my secret in my professional arena but there was no speed limit between me and her at the end of the day. There was an Arkansas State trooper with a $325 ticket for me that said otherwise but I literally felt I had no choice. I practically had to break the sound barrier getting home in time because of that trooper. Just how long does it take to write a ticket for Pete's sake?

If depression hasn't been a significant part of your experience in life so far, noticing the signs of depression may be a little harder. Everyone has down days. That is inevitable because we exist as humans in an imperfect reality. The difficulty is when the down days are lingering, and the up days are a distant memory. Knowing the signs of depression may be helpful for those like me who are used to pushing past and ignoring what they feel.

The signs and symptoms of depression are very much the same for all types, but situational depression related to the grief process may be more noticeable as a change to one's usual nature. Here's what it might feel like:

❖ Persistent feelings of hopelessness or pessimism especially when this isn't how you normally felt before cancer.

❖ Feelings of guilt, worthlessness, or helplessness as your mortality is being threatened.

❖ Irritability, especially at small things that would have never bothered you before.

❖ Decreased energy or fatigue. This is a tough one because cancer treatment alone can make you feel burned out.

❖ Loss of interest or pleasure in hobbies and activities or having lost the joy of doing things you still can do.

❖ Moving or talking with agitation or moving abnormally slowly. This is harder to notice in yourself, but others may mention it to you.

❖ Difficulty making decisions, memory problems, or inability to concentrate which feels like the normal bargaining phase! Suspect depression if the clouds never seem to lift.

❖ Difficulty sleeping, staying asleep, or sleeping too much. Recovery needs adequate sleep but sleep disturbances due to depression seem like any sleep you get isn't enough.

❖ Appetite or weight changes. Many weight changes can be attributed to chemotherapy or hormonal therapy. Eating changes due to depression may not be as obvious. However, radical weight changes can cause additional emotional problems.

❖ Pain, headaches, or digestive issues without a clear physical cause that do not get better with treatment. The first action for this is to talk to your medical health provider. It can get tricky to add in other vitamins, herbs, over-the-counter meds, or other treatment modalities without working with your medical provider.

❖ Thoughts of death, suicide, or self-harm. Please get help. Don't hold these feelings on your own.

If any of the above resonates with how you are feeling, you are not alone. You are not broken, deficient, or going about your life in the wrong way. It's okay to need help. It takes strength to acknowledge what you feel and even more to reach out for help.

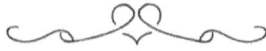

Getting through the initial trials of breast cancer seemed easier because of the support of my friends and family. It was like having love surround me at my toughest time. I had a small but very appreciated cheerleading squad.

But then I got past chemo and treatments. My hair grew back, and my face no longer was the color of death. My husband stopped being quite so helpful around the house, grateful to give up some of his caregiver duties. A relative remarked that it was all behind me now so I "should just move on." People's priorities reverted to surviving their own daily challenges and I was alone. I was supposed to feel better, but I didn't. I was more scared of never feeling myself again, never being completely free of cancer because I would always have the threat of reoccurrence looming. This was the time I needed help the most.

Cancer happened once. What's to say that it can't come back? And if it does, what will that mean for my life? My personal crystal ball wasn't speaking to me no matter how hard I shake it. I don't know the future or how I will live the rest of my life much less how I will die. I do know that when I focus my attention on what might happen, I can't see what is true right now. Generally, if I stay present in the moment, I'm usually safe and can handle whatever I'm dealing with. It's the unknown that gets me tied into a knot of tension without even realizing that it is happening. That tension became chronic and dogged my every waking moment, stealing my joy for life.

Thankfully, my chemo experience was energetically draining enough that I didn't have the ability to worry about the future because getting through the day was all I could do. Those fears tended to creep in later when I let them. I was a couple of years out from chemo when I finally realized I felt like crap mentally, spiritually, and physically. My annual oncology appointment was coming up, so I did the smart thing and decided to talk to my oncologist, Dr. Makhoul, about it. He listened but didn't prescribe me any medications nor give me advice. He simply asked me to think of a way to put it on paper, all the goodness I could think of that helped me so far.

In all honesty, I did that inner eye roll thing because I didn't want to be rude. But it got me to thinking. I thought about my husband doing his best to clean up the results of my vertigo and the revolving toilet that I tried to throw up in. I remembered my first shower after my mastectomy. My husband stood at the shower door holding my drains as I sobbed in pain, his eyes full of concern. I thought of Maggie, my beloved canine beacon of unconditional compassion, my friends, family, plates of food that magically found their way to my kitchen table, and even Dr. Makhoul, who was with me during the darkest days of my life. I imagined them as interwoven threads of love blanketing my shoulders, giving me the strength to release all the pain, fear, and isolation cancer had brought me.

One stumbling block to dealing with dark days is the push to think that it could be worse or other people have it worse than you. I've brought this up before, but it bears repeating. Variations of a famous quote that has been credited to many different sources goes something like, "I cried because I had no shoes until I met a man with no feet." There will always be someone who has it worse. That doesn't mean that what you and I go through on a daily basis is trivial. What we feel is real to us and to shame ourselves into denying what we feel because it could be worse is, in my opinion, one of the most disempowering things we can allow to happen. I have met several women who have had Stage 0 breast cancer and felt guilty or refused to claim to have had the trauma of getting breast cancer because it wasn't more advanced. Stage 0 breast cancer or carcinoma in situ means cancer that hasn't moved from the original place and after removal, doesn't always require further treatment. It's still cancer. If you honestly feel it was just a "cancer scare," that's great but if the breast cancer diagnosis rocked you to the core even for a short time, honor what you feel and have gone through. Stage 0 through Stage 4 is still cancer, and no matter your staging, you have experienced trauma.

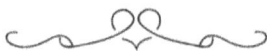

⌒◡◡◡◡⌒

Soon after my reconstruction, I sought out some breast cancer forums on the American Cancer Society website. This was pre-Facebook group era. I was hoping to find out if all the pain, itchiness, and ugliness of my reconstruction was across the board typical, so I posted a question to the members. I got one response.

"Don't you think you might have a problem with vanity?"

I reeled in shock as if I had been slapped right through that webpage. Then I realized I was on a forum for lifers. All these women were Stage 4 and supporting each other in their end stages of life. Their priorities were different. That doesn't mean I didn't have a right to how I felt about my reconstruction. I was just in the wrong group.

What I needed then and did not receive was support for the emotional devastation I was feeling. Although there are cancer centers (for example the Cancer Treatment Centers of America), that address emotional and behavioral needs, this support should be available to everyone experiencing cancer. Getting help should be offered up front and not later when things have gotten well out of hand.

Too many people have been raised to believe they aren't good enough as they are. They spend much of their life comparing themselves to some perceived ideal, an impossible and unattainable goal. Lots of media images of depression have people holding masks of different emotions with their true expressions hiding behind them. The effort to present as someone you are not makes it hard to even recognize what you really feel. Cancer, chemo, surgeries, and medications can drain your energy, leaving you unable to hold up your mask. If you were holding the mask to protect yourself from not being accepted by others, all the changes to your body and soul because of cancer will make lowering that mask feel unsafe. You no longer have the energy to try to be someone you are not, but it is too dangerous to be yourself.

We are given signals that we must hide who we truly are and pretend to be who we are not to gain acceptance. We are pushed to smile and be happy, think of others, shame ourselves for feeling low, wonder what the heck is wrong with ourselves, or even medicate ourselves to keep from feeling anything at all. There is a huge pressure to be someone we are not. The drive to fit in is deeply embedded in our survival.

The more we try to fake a smile or shame ourselves for being depressed, the harder and longer it keeps us entrenched in its drama. Sometimes, when we are at our lowest, we are willing to go inside seeking to create a way to bring back some beauty into our lives. What if the lowest times in a person's life are the darkest days before dawn? What if we stopped fighting ourselves because of depression and instead, looked for something worthwhile about what we are experiencing? What if we valued our time of inner reflection as an exploration of what is and what can be? What if depression is a sign that there are things in our lives that no longer serve us and we need to release? What if it is a sign that we are trying too hard to be what other people expect of us?

When you are going through the trauma of cancer and possibly the chemotherapy, radiological, or surgical ramifications of cancer, you may not have the energy to be strong for everyone else. Children tend to absorb your sadness which makes them feel unsafe and somehow responsible, so mothers and grandmothers tend to hide their feelings to protect them. Children simply cannot process the emotional upheaval you may be going through. It is only natural to want to shield them from your true feelings and fears. Other family and friends may struggle to process what you are going through, also. Then your battle gets worse. You end up trying to manage the normal, predictable depression of this phase as well as the needs and reactions of everyone around you.

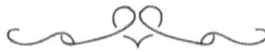

I knew I was going to lose my hair. My oncologist told me not to shave my head too early because some people don't lose their hair completely. He said it may just become thin in places. I don't know if he was just being kind, but my hair was already thin in places. I have really thin, straight, wispy hair on my best days. I challenge any baby to a who-has-the-thinnest-baby-soft-hair competition.

Much of my youth was uselessly spent dreaming of getting struck by lightning where my hair would be burned off but magically grows back in lush, thick, luxuriously wavy, maybe even curly hair that flows down my back straining my little neck under the weight. Fortunately, I acquired a little common sense over my lifetime and stopped wishing to get struck by lightning, but I still held out a tiny bit of hope that I would wake up one day with different hair. I had a few people tell me they knew someone who went through chemo and lost their hair only for it to grow back curly and gorgeous. At the time, this didn't really factor in as being important to me because I was still freaked out about having to start chemo. It felt like I had about eight billion years of challenges to get through before I would be concerned about growing any-thing back on my head.

Just to be the prepared-for-anything gal, I went to the Little Rock office of the American Cancer Society. I was told I could pick out a wig to use later if I were to need it. I was willing to get a wig, but I kept telling myself I wasn't going to need it. It seemed I was getting pretty good at lying to myself. However, if you aren't totally invested in getting a decent wig, you tend to do exactly what I did. I somehow managed to find the ugliest, rattiest wig in the bin.

My first mistake was taking my husband to help me pick it out. He was still as shell-shocked as I was and he was so afraid of hurting my feelings that, had I put a bale of hay on my head, he would have said I looked just fine. The wigs were in big bins like you would find in a thrift store and were full of limp, hairy blobs waiting to be adopted. They were at least roughly grouped according to color so I could easily pass over the bins of brunette and red wigs on my way to the blonde ones. Everyone must either be or want to be a blonde because the sheer number of blonde wigs was staggering. I felt sorry for the brunettes of the world because they had slim pickings.

I gingerly picked up a wig off the top of the pile and put it on. My husband said I looked lovely. I have to take his word for it because I couldn't see out of the curtain of bangs that fell across my chin. I was doing a good imitation of the pop singer Sia with that wig. I pulled it off and tossed it back in the bin. I have never been a garage sale fan. Going butt up, digging through boxes and bins for some hidden treasure was never my life's goal so I wasn't getting very far looking for a wig. I picked up a second wig and jammed it on my head and looked at my husband. Come to think of it, surely there was a mirror in that joint, but I don't think I saw one. This time he didn't say anything, so I jerked the offending hairy blob off my head and tossed it back in the bin.

By then, I was done. I surveyed the jumbled mass of wigs with desperation knowing I couldn't leave without picking out one of them. Snatching up another, I mashed that maligned wig on my head with a vengeance. I picked a wig; now let me out of here. I signed some kind of form and left with my prized possession as fast as I could. Later that evening in the privacy of my bathroom, I tried the wig on again. It wasn't too bad. It would be just fine... if I were joining a circus freak show or maybe wanting to look like the Living Dead. I looked like I had been struck by lightning. I pushed the front of the wig up on my forehead a bit and felt some crunchy ends. I pulled it off and looked closely at it. The last poor soul that had this wig had used a curling iron to try to control the spiky wads of hair that jutted out where bangs should be. That works for real hair, but this was plastic fake hair. The bangs were melted into crispy, knobby ends. Only I could pick out a wig that had melted off bangs. No wonder I could see out from under them.

After I ended up losing my hair, I took the wig out of the closet where I had shoved it, shook it a few times and put it on. It seemed a bit loose. I could tell this by the fact that I swiveled my head left really fast, and the wig never moved. I was now looking through the side of the wig. I imagined walking down a street and a gust of wind *blowing my wig off, and me, in all my bald glory, chasing after my miniature, blonde tumbleweed.*

I have a little head. I didn't know that until then, but I should have been looking at youth-sized wigs. (Passing thought here but I hope my head size isn't directly proportional to my IQ because it would mean my brothers were right about me all along.) Getting back to the world of wigs, I learned that when you try a wig on while you still have hair you get a false estimation of fit because your hair is taking up room. It is just not going to fit the same—even with wispy hair. Also, you will need one of those little caps to wear under the wig to help hold it on because without hair, your head is a little slick. Without something like the cap, go out on a windy day and you might end up chasing your own miniature tumbleweed.

My heart sank every time I tried that wig on my sparsely fuzzy head. Since wearing a wig wasn't for me, I learned how to use scarves instead. I still held out hope that my hair would grow back curly but nope, it is as straight, fine, and baby soft as ever. At least I can still win that baby hair competition.

There are tons of euphemisms and advice for dealing with depression and I refuse to inflict them on anyone. Therefore, I can only address what I found that helped me. First of all, I stopped fighting it. Not that I wallowed in my depression, but I stopped denying its presence; I no longer tried to hide it or cover it up with a bunch of other activity.

Seriously, trying to control depression is like holding a beach ball under the waves. The nanosecond your grip slips, that sucker is shooting skyward like a rocket, spraying water everywhere. It's exhausting.

There are famous quotes that tell us that where we focus our attention is where we place our energy and then that grows stronger in our lives. I was afraid to acknowledge my depression because I was afraid it would make it worse. However, there is a fine line between choosing to avoid what we feel and forcing ourselves to feel something else. We can distract ourselves for a time but until we accept ourselves and our dark times, seeing the light remains a struggle.

Choosing to not fight my depression wasn't surrendering to it. I realized I had an internal limit to how deeply I wanted to feel into it before I was done. I had to trust myself that even though I was experiencing depression, I was not my depression. There is infinite power in words. We often say I am sad, depressed, or angry. That is effectively saying that we *are* that emotion. When we say we are what we feel, we are no longer empowered to make changes. Who we are is harder to change than what we feel. We are not the emotions; we feel emotions. Accepting ourselves without judgment even when we feel depressed is the first step to kicking it to the curb. Maybe we change the phrase to "I feel depressed."

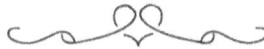

During the days when I was just finishing up chemo and growing fuzz on my head again, we had a wonderful prosthetics and post-mastectomy apparel shop in my hometown of Russellville, AR called Pink Ribbon Boutique, Inc. There were lovely ladies who always greeted me with huge smiles of welcome and were so helpful to help me normalize my appearance with undergarments that disguised my architectural aberrations. Even though the Pink Ribbon Boutique, Inc. ultimately moved to a new location with new management, having such a wonderfully supportive shop run by caring people who help breast

cancer veterans maximize their individualized needs was invaluable to me.

One day while shopping there, Carolyn, the shop owner, beckoned me to a corner to sit where she asked me to consider being part of their fundraiser for breast cancer awareness. They were putting together a calendar high-lighting twelve women and their stories. It sounded pretty wonderful, but you have to know that I had recently watched a movie about older ladies making a leukemia fundraiser calendar in the UK, Calendar Girls (2003). They were photographed in the nude with items artistically hiding what should not be seen.

Was she wanting me to embrace my Frankenboobs and do a nude photo shoot for breast cancer awareness? I still choose to blame chemo for giving me the mental acuity of a snail, but alarms in my head were screaming so loud I couldn't think. With my mouth gaping like a goldfish, I stared at her so long she probably wondered about my mental health. She was right to wonder. I finally stuttered out the question if it was to be in the nude.

Why on earth she thought it was so funny that she nearly fell off her chair and peed her pants is beyond me. It was a perfectly reasonable question to ask. At least it sounded that way in my head. Turns out that I got to keep covered and Maggie, my canine constant companion, was in the photo, too. We were Ms. November with our story of how we got through chemo side by side. I got a makeover complete with fake eyelashes that lifted my spirits tremendously. Maggie ended up stealing the limelight of our photo shoot and made it all about her doggie joy, which was fine with me. However, we would have probably raised more money had Maggie been artistically hiding my nude chest, but nobody listens to me. Just saying.

Here are some things I tried that did seem to reduce the intensity of situational depression and ease my passage through this phase:

Walking helped me. I had a daily walking habit for as long as I can remember. It was my preferred method of exercise in the past because I could get outside and walk with my dogs. Getting to enjoy the world through their excitement was one of the best parts of my day. When I moved from back hills of Arkansas to relative civilization in 2008, I had only Maggie with me to walk the neighborhood instead of isolated dirt roads. We thrived on those walks.

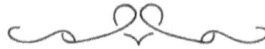

When chemo drained my energy to zero, I wanted to sit on my couch when I was tired of lying down. Maggie and I argued about going for walks often. She won most of those arguments since she had an uncannily accurate intuition as to my ability to walk on a particular day. Just because I could put one foot in front of the other in a rhythmical pattern didn't necessarily mean I wanted to do so. That is what we argued the most about. At the end of the day, I was glad my twenty-pound tyrant won. Even though my joints hurt to walk, I had no energy, and I complained most of the way, I always felt better.

Companionship helps. Maggie was my constant companion, but our one-sided conversations sometimes weren't enough. My husband worked and was great company when he got home, but I needed girl talk. Most of the time, I didn't have the energy for prolonged conversations so a text from a friend saying "I'm thinking of you" was the perfect connection. Getting a card in the mail gave me joy that lasted for days. I didn't feel forgotten. I reached out when I needed a friend, and I would find a lifeline.

Although some people feel hesitant to tell someone going through cancer treatment about their own little life issues, that is exactly what we need to hear sometimes. Putting aside the cancer world for a few minutes is restoring whether the conversation is about a husband throwing his dirty underwear in the general vicinity of a hamper or better yet, a bit of innocuous gossip. Cancer was probably my least favorite topic for conversation. Responding to how I was feeling ran a close second. The important thing is to not isolate yourself. That gets too lonely.

Sleep is great. Restorative sleep is priceless. And no, all sleep is not the same. Going through the stress of a cancer diagnosis changes hormonal levels. Cortisol, which is the main stress hormone, regulates a lot of things in the body such as inflamemation levels, blood pressure, blood sugar, and sleep/wake cycles. The purpose is to help the body to respond to normal stress and danger. When working correctly, the levels fluctuate throughout the day according to your needs. Major, prolonged stress and pain blow normal cortisol levels out of the water. If you have to take steroids (man-made cortisol) in preparation for chemotherapy, the levels get even further out of whack.

If cortisol levels are too high, you struggle to shut your brain up long enough to fall asleep. High cortisol levels also make you crave sugar and fat, so weight gain becomes a concern. It also affects blood sugar and increases the risk for diabetes as well as making existing diabetes harder to control. Increased cortisol levels are needed to reduce pain and inflammation and are a vital part of chemotherapy. Lower cortisol levels can make you feel exhausted no matter how many hours of sleep you get. With all the other health issues that happen because of cancer treatment, it can get overwhelming. It can feel like playing the game Whack-A-Mole.

Anything you can do to help yourself get good sleep is important. Try not to stay up too late past your normal circadian rhythm. Baths are soothing if you don't have any physical reasons not to submerge in water. Limiting screen time in the evenings and turning them off entirely an hour before bedtime is good. I had to move my phone and iPad into another room to get myself to stop reaching for them. I was worse than a three-year-old not wanting to nap because I would lie down then hop up immediately to go look something up or scroll social media. During the day, I could keep my mind occupied enough to not focus on my problems but those few moments before falling asleep were sheer torture because of the fears crowding in. In an attempt to soothe my anxiety and paralyze my brain, I rotated through several games on my iPad until I was exhausted enough to fall asleep. All those games I played kept me awake until the early hours of the morning, never letting me get enough healing rest.

Try starting a new pastime or hobby. That is if you have the energy to do so. Starting something new or renewing a past hobby gives you a creative outlet for what you are feeling.

Set realistic goals. You may have gotten to this point in the blink of an eye but set yourself up for success by giving yourself all the time you need to recover. Goals give your brain a direction to focus, where to go. Small, achievable goals give you micro-wins you can celebrate. I couldn't walk my previous three miles but when I set a goal for the end of my street and made it, I was just as proud of myself.

Join a support group. Not all support groups are the same. When I was going through treatment, the support groups I knew were available promoted things to do to make myself feel better like makeup and finding wigs. Facebook is good for community, but a lot of misinformation can go rampant. The right kind of support group would be where a person can feel supported in a non-judgmental way and address the major issues the trauma of breast cancer brings up.

This is where the dream of my heart lies. I hope to see more professionally led support groups that preferably use energy medicine techniques such as Emotional Freedom Techniques (EFT) available free or at an absurdly low cost to the participant. Talk therapy is not always enough. Emotional health is as important and vital as physical health. We can't address one without the other. Cancer means trauma and few have access to help to manage that trauma. I needed help and I believe we all need and deserve that help. I hope to see a movement in providing the emotional and psychological help for every person experiencing breast cancer. Cancer support groups should be designed to help with the losses of cancer and not just information about where to find a free wig.

Pot of Gold at the End of the Rainbow: Acceptance

For after all, the best thing one can do when it is raining is to let it rain.

Henry Wadsworth Longfellow

W hy is this happening to ME? What did I do wrong? Was there something so inherently wrong with me that God or the Universe or someone was punishing me for some mistake I didn't know I made? Did I drink from too many BPA toxic bottles? Did I hurt someone and karma was coming to bite me? Was it the pesticides in my food? Did I just win the elimination lottery? I was told that my cancer is because of anger turned inward, so is my cancer my fault? Why did God let this happen to me? Why won't someone answer me?

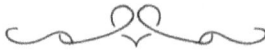

One of the first things I asked my oncologist Dr. Makhoul, one of the most compassionate healers I've encountered, when I got diagnosed with breast cancer was why did this happen to me? He was gentle but quick to tell me not to ask why because there is no answer. He hoped that I wouldn't torture myself with an unanswerable question. With all due respect, a lot of good that did. I was consumed with worry, yet I felt I was somehow wrong to ask.

I heard the phrase "I don't ask why me, but why not me?" Bless my chemo-riddled brain, but I could never understand what that meant. Did asking why mean I was so arrogant that I believed I couldn't or shouldn't get cancer? That one hits a bit too close to home, but I still don't know about the why not me part. Is that to be how I'm supposed to think about getting cancer to prove my humility? Is it to demonstrate that fate is in control, and I don't have the right to question it?

No matter how hard I worked, I couldn't stop trying to figure out how breast cancer happened to me. I thought that if I could figure out why I got cancer, not only could I avoid whatever that was in the future so it doesn't come back, but also maybe I could find acceptance. Since I wasn't supposed to question why or what I did to get cancer, maybe I was just supposed to chalk it up to the luck of the draw. I was the ant on the sidewalk that got stepped on. At least that is what it felt like. How was I supposed to accept that with grace?

Feeling like I was not allowed to ask, therefore never finding a logical reason it happened, meant I could spend the rest of my life searching for a meaning, a purpose that made having cancer okay. Maybe it happened because I was too repressed or wasn't taking care of myself as I should. Maybe cancer was my wake-up call, my gift to point out all the ways I was not doing something right. Some gift.

Acceptance, in theory, sounds like nirvana so I fought like hell to obtain that elusive sense of peace. The harder I fought, driving myself crazy to find a reason or the so-called gift in my cancer, the more evasive it became. I clearly didn't know what acceptance really meant. All I knew was that I had to find it, whatever it was.

The End Game or Not

Isn't acceptance supposed to be the pot of gold at the end of the rainbow, a reward for getting through all the phases of grief? At least that is what I was led to believe. Only that's not how it worked out for me. It wasn't the end game. I didn't get through all the tests of life and to a point that I never had another problem with having had cancer. It would seem that I was doing great, and another aspect of cancer would rear its ugly head and bam, I would be starting over again. The first few times I stumbled through all these phases and got to the point that I wasn't fighting it anymore, I thought I was done. My depression lifted and I felt I had moved on. Then, the peripheral crap that comes with having experienced cancer would rise up and make me doubt I got anywhere at all.

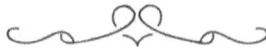

A few years after going through chemotherapy, I was back at the hospital for an X-ray of my chest for some reason that I can't remember now. It showed a small, suspicious area in my sternum and required follow up with an MRI. Suddenly, all that I had been through was back in my face. All the shock, fears, and emotional turmoil were like they had never left.

Sure, I knew there were always going to be routine exams, tests, and follow up in my future but they weren't supposed to actually find anything! This was not supposed to happen! Eventually, everything turned out okay. The suspicious area couldn't be found on the MRI but that was well after I rode that cancer roller coaster of fear one more time.

It's incredibly hard to let something just be. The desire to find some reason behind all that we go through is so pervasive, keeping us focused on the pain and unfairness of what is happening. Looking for answers to every situation and question in our lives can get crazy making. Questions like *How I am going to deal with this?* or *Why did this happen?* keep us focused on what went wrong. Our brains are driven to find answers to our questions, but the purpose isn't to punish us for where we screwed up in life. Our primitive, reactive, lizard brains are there to protect us at all costs. The drive to find answers is just a way for the brain to think up all the ways something might have happened so we can avoid repeating it in the future. It just feels like punishment if we don't understand what ol' lizard brain is doing. Before I could really understand any part of this phase, I had to look at what I discovered that acceptance isn't.

Acceptance isn't finding the right answer. It also isn't controlling the brain into stopping the questions from coming up. It is more like no longer needing the answer. It is totally okay to wonder why things happen. It isn't in our best interests to rationalize, settle for explanations that deplete us or come up with possibilities just for the sake of having somewhere to pin the responsibility. It also doesn't serve us to have something or someone to blame. It's okay to wonder why I got cancer and it's okay that I'll never know why.

Acceptance isn't forgetting. I once thought that if I just quit fighting it and accepted that my life would never be the same, I could go back to a slightly different version of life where I could forget I had breast cancer. I knew in the back of my mind that I wouldn't really be able to forget but maybe I would get to a point where I would be so busy that my breast cancer wouldn't be in my face every day. This was really denial masquerading as acceptance. I was still trying to figure out a way that breast cancer wouldn't be a part of my life.

Acceptance isn't giving up the fight. Breast cancer sucks. Change the first letter of *sucks* to an *f* and that is more like what I experienced. I fought back hard with all I had and in many ways that was a good thing. It never got me the results I thought I wanted but I got results. I thought I could fight back and defeat cancer. I won many battles but walked away with battle scars, trauma, and PTSD. If acceptance means giving up the fight and allowing breast cancer to have at me with both fists, I couldn't do that. I thought I needed my anger to fuel me through winning. I thought that once I'd won the battle, I would have a sense of acceptance. I could tell myself that cancer came and took but I ultimately won therefore I can accept that it all happened. Only I never really felt I won. I couldn't make cancer do what my heart wanted, which was to go back in time and have it never happen.

We should never give up the fight to make things better for ourselves. We just don't have to fight all the unseen forces behind why breast cancer happened in the first place. Keep fighting to focus on what is gained, not what was lost.

Acceptance isn't making rationalizations. I tried to find some profound meaning around my getting cancer because that would give a purpose to my experience. A lot of people say that getting cancer was a huge wake-up call to areas of their lives that needed healing. Once they acknowledged that and made those changes, they were in a state of peace and acceptance. That is a beautiful way to approach the breast cancer experience. Congratulations to all who are able to do so, but I wasn't one of them.

If I needed such a devastating, life-altering, wake-up call to point out where I screwed up so miserably and this is what it takes to straighten me out, I must be flawed to the core. I hoped that when I decided my cancer was a necessary evil, I would be in a state of acceptance. It would be okay that I got cancer because I've learned my lesson now. Even though the worst that can happen did, I don't have to be ashamed because I've handled it so well. *I took my punishment, served my sentence with valor. See how well I have done?* This was me bargaining with my experience to find a way I could accept it.

Acceptance isn't saying I'm a failure. To accept that cancer came in a blaze of hellish fury and took more than its fair share of my body and life doesn't mean I was defeated. Acceptance doesn't mean believing that I suck so badly that I needed cancer to salvage me. If I gave up and believed the fear in my heart that I was not good enough to have a life untouched by cancer, the darkness of depression would have overtaken me. Acceptance of what is happening isn't a judgment of me or what I have done. Instead, it is making the conscious effort to step aside from all judgment and beliefs around my breast cancer and just be who I am at heart.

Acceptance is not really about accepting having cancer but accepting who we are as well as who we've become as a result of experiencing our cancers. My battle with acceptance of my cancer was rooted in my belief that it was just another measure of proof that I did not deserve to live. I spent many years trying to figure out the meaning of my cancer only to realize that was a useless feat. The meaning of my life is much more than cancer.

After my breast cancer diagnosis, I tried all the tricks and experienced all the work of trying to mentally figure a way to manage my cancer. I went through the emotional roller coasters in reaction to the devastation of cancer. It was natural for me to wonder why cancer happens but all this fight to understand why is a waste of precious energy that someone going through cancer and treatment doesn't have to spare. That is why Dr. Makhoul wanted me not to ask why. He had no answers, but he knew that keeping me focused on what I did wrong would steal my strength for getting through the challenges facing me in the moment. There is nothing that can be done to alter the basic facts we cannot control. But we can choose to control how we react to what cancer has done to us. Once we accept that we can only control how we react and what we allow to define us as individuals, we can then stop allowing cancer to control us. No matter what percentage we have of prognosis for survival, we can choose to be 100 percent alive.

Breast cancer didn't happen to me, or for me, or because of me. It happened with me. As with any life challenge, I get to choose how I want to live my life and what defines me. I won't allow that definition to be breast cancer. Instead, it will be the stronger version of me as a result of what I've gone through because of breast cancer.

Acceptance is about appreciating the new priorities for living and newfound strengths we see inside ourselves. As women in general, we have mastered the art of putting ourselves last. Most of us strive to prove our worth by what we do, and society encourages us to martyr ourselves for the sake of others. Martyrdom has reached toxic levels because we are conditioned to believe we should care for others at the expense of ourselves. That whole "put your oxygen mask on first" has a good point. You can't care for others when you are dead.

There is a compelling need for many of us to try to prove our value because not everyone feels an inherent sense of self-worth. Since it is not easily felt and many have had life experiences that challenged our self-worth, we burn ourselves out trying to build some evidence of value to our existence. Acceptance tells us that what we can or can't do now because of cancer has no bearing on our worth as human beings. Our value stems from who we are, not what we do to earn it. Just because we struggle to feel our value doesn't mean we don't have any. We have value because we exist.

Acceptance is about appreciation and gratitude. I've read from many sources that gratitude is what we should strive for in enlightenment. Religions base much doctrine on gratitude for all things which in theory sounds really nice. It's not that easy to actually accomplish. Gratitude is easy with a full belly and money in your pocket. It gets a little tricky with your head in a waste-basket dry heaving or dealing with the aftermath of losing your job or partner. Still a worthy goal but along with the whole concept of acceptance, gratitude is a minefield of misinterpretations.

The term *gratitude* is provoking or triggering for some. If you have ever been on the receiving end of a conversation that contained, "You should be grateful..." "You ungrateful little..." then gratitude gets perceived as just another way you don't measure up. Gratitude becomes another stick to be beaten with. That's why I prefer to use the term *appreciate*. And that's why acceptance is so important. Once we are able to accept what is and stop trying to make it what we want it to be, we have more energy to appreciate what we have gained, not lost, because of cancer.

Acceptance is about being better able to stay present in the moment.

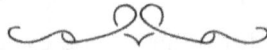

For as long as I can remember, I've had negative thought loops running in my head, which make it nearly impossible to stay present in the moment. I couldn't let go of distressing thoughts, events, possibilities, or worry about something I did or didn't do. Then I was worried that something ugly might happen as a result. Sometimes the thoughts would be like a review of everything I did or said to see if I made a mistake but sometimes it was clearly abusive criticism, only I was my own bully.

I had done quite a bit of study, research, and work trying to get rid of that negative self-talk, but I failed miserably. I was told to recognize and challenge those thoughts, be my own best friend, and focus on positive things. Focus on the present, they said, and if that doesn't work, seek professional help. Fat lot of good that did for me. I couldn't stay present in the moment because I was too busy worrying about screwing up and beating myself up for not being perfect. Professional help would have been wonderful, but I felt it wasn't an option for me.

One night about 3 a.m., I was startled awake. I had an overwhelming sense that I was in mortal danger. I lay as still as I could, my heart pounding like a drum as I listened for sounds of an intruder. Nothing but the soft breathing of my husband sleeping beside me came to my ears, so I tried to relax. Immediately, my mind started to assess all that I had done the day before for things that I may have done wrong or should have done but didn't. It was my inner critic, my negative self-talk. the critical accounting of everything I am and do, never missing an opportunity to drag me down.

As I lay quietly in bed that night, praying to be able to go back to sleep even though I knew it was a losing battle, I started thinking about EFT which shows that many of our coping skills were developed as a result of experiences from our childhoods. I've asked many clients that I facilitated with EFT how long they felt a certain way, so I asked myself, How long I have had my inner critic tormenting me? *And the answer was,* As long as I can remember. *As a child, there was never a time I felt safe. I was always on guard for my mother's moods. Although I wasn't physically abused, I never knew when I would be in trouble. I desperately tried to follow the rules, but the rules were always changing. I could do something fifty times and the fifty-first time, she would be towering over me screaming, her eyes blazing with anger. I was a kid and did not have the capacity to understand I wasn't the problem, just the unfortunate and easiest target of an overwhelmed parent. I took it personally. Her anger taught me that I wasn't good enough and no matter how hard I worked to prove my value to her, I would never make it.*

I became hypervigilant for any signs that I could be attacked which meant analyzing everything I did and didn't do. Being punished for my mistakes was to be expected, but I also had a fear of being attacked for something not in my control. This was an intense fear about the rules that kept changing without notice. As time went on, that fear evolved into a constant stream of self-criticism in the form of a negative thought loop.

Lying quietly beside my sleeping husband willing myself to fall asleep, an image of a child formed in my mind. She was about five years old, her long, stringy, blond hair flowing over her thin shoulders. As she looked up toward some unseen malevolent force, her blue eyes welled with tears threatening to spill down her cheeks. She was confused, frightened, and desperate to feel loved. That little girl was me.

I watched as she turned to me and drew close to whisper in my ear. She whispered that we needed to look over everything I had done, said, or not done to see if there was anything I could be attacked over. She wanted me to look for anything possibly wrong so I could avoid doing that again. That's when it hit me. The voice of my inner critic that I thought was abject condemnation spewing proof that I terminally suck was really the voice of a terrified little girl trying to prevent me from doing anything that might get me screamed at. My inner critic is the voice of a child trying to protect me in the only way she knows how. No wonder I couldn't override that voice.

My husband was very used to me always asking a vague, "Is it going to be okay?" He learned early in our marriage that this wasn't something he could tease me about or not take seriously. I needed him to tell me it was going to be okay. Some days, I must have asked him too many times to count but it never changed the way I felt. I kept asking. Knowing the anxiety was that little girl inside of me still seeking reassurance, I realized I could do that for myself. As I told my inner child that I had this and it was going to be okay, I could handle any mistakes I made, that familiar feeling of dread and anxiety slipped away. I finally was able to believe it myself. A sense of peace settled over me like I've never known before, and I fell back asleep.

I made peace with my past and my negative self-talk with the help of EFT. As I did, I learned to stop fighting negative self-talk and, instead, to comfort that part of me that was so scared back then. I finally realized that my cancer wasn't my punishment for being me. I hadn't done anything wrong. Then I listened for the loop, but it was gone. For the first time I can remember, I felt safe.

———————

Silencing negative self-talk loops means living in the present moment, not worrying about the past or what might happen in the future. It promotes feeling safer and bringing more happiness. It helps us to enjoy what is happening now and to live for today. By accepting and staying present without the internal bullying, we are able to reduce stress and decrease the impact of stress on our health, helping us handle pain more effectively, improve our ability to cope, and make room for more joy. We could all use more of that.

There is no clear road map to acceptance. My trying to translate all I could gather around the topic of acceptance is like nailing Jell-O to a tree. There is no one book, lecture, pill, or illicit substance that will get us from point A to point B without doing some serious internal reflection. If acceptance were that easy or generic, there wouldn't be so many people in the world grappling with grief and acceptance for a vast array of reasons. Acceptance is as unique and individual as each one of us. The funny part is that true acceptance happens when you are busy getting on with living life fully.

Perhaps the truth about acceptance is so easy that we can't believe it. Maybe acceptance is really self-acceptance. It's not the reward at the end of a long race with cancer but simply loving and accepting yourself as you are today, warts and all. Loving and accepting ourselves as we are right now may sound simple, but the hardest thing we ever try to do. It also may be the most necessary thing we ever attempt.

I believe true acceptance is more of a day-to-day, fluid state of being with what is. Some days are good, and some days suck big time. It has less to do with your emotions and more with how you choose to feel. Acceptance grows as you are able to stop judging yourself for getting—and getting through—cancer. For me, acceptance came as I learned to accept myself for who I am, which is a day-to-day process, too. Some days will suck but the future looks pretty promising.

I can accept that.

To Speak or Not to Speak:
That Is the Question

The amazing truth about the human tongue: It
takes three years to learn how to use it, but it takes
a lifetime to learn when and where to use it.

Anonymous

Maybe you have been the recipient of some very unfortunate, unwelcome advice about how you should feel or what you should do or not do. Telling someone you have breast cancer is awkward at best and downright painful at others. Inevitably, vague offers of help come from well-meaning people who simply are stunned and do not know how to respond in the best way. When you are still mired in your grief process, it is easy to take some of the advice or empty offers for help personally and not in the spirit that the person intended. If you have been conditioned to always think of the other person, the fact that they could say such hurtful, or at least unhelpful things, is hard to understand. This section doesn't include the truly malicious or uncaring people out there. They do not deserve to be in your breathing space in the first place.

It is my hope and purpose in this section to help guide the general public to know what to say and bring awareness to the impact of misspoken words. Additionally, I want to let all of us know we are not alone in what hurtful things have been said to us in the past. Having to deal with clumsy or hurtful remarks during a time that you are working your way through the phases of grief around your cancer diagnosis is tough. It's not a great time to navigate all the nuances of social interactions.

Dealing with insensitive or hurtful people may be easy for some, so this is for the ones (like me) who struggle with confrontation. Acknowledging your feelings and the right to *have* your feelings is important. Insensitive remarks do hurt, and it is okay to feel hurt or angry in the moment no matter how good the intentions of the speaker are. On the other hand, just trying to think of the other person only helps so much. As women, we are typically masters at putting others before ourselves. If we totally understand it is okay to have boundaries and that we can love ourselves enough to calmly hold those boundaries, what people inadvertently say can no longer harm us.

I recently polled a Facebook group of breast cancer veterans for things that were said to them that didn't land with joy. I also asked what they wish they would have heard. There were common themes, so I wanted to put them here so you would know you aren't alone if you are the recipient of one or more. For those readers who aren't personally facing breast cancer, please keep reading. There are some verbal landmines that can be avoided. I'm using their words with little editing.

"You can get a pink wig now."

"You can name your wigs like Moira on *Schitt's Creek*."

There really isn't any upside to losing all your hair. Especially if you don't get a choice in the matter. A few actresses caused media uproar after shaving their heads because of some emotional trauma. There also was a COVID 2020 movement of freedom by shaving your head and losing the peer pressure to maintain a certain appearance of femininity or in avoidance of heteronormativity. I applaud the women who choose to do so despite peer pressure and the blowback of people's reactions.

Your hair represents the first impression of your identity to the public which in turn can impact how you feel about yourself. If your hair is great, you feel better about yourself. Bad hair days are often felt as days where nothing goes right. The texture, thickness, color, and style all are incredibly important to our self-esteem. Losing your hair also announces to the world that you are going through cancer treatment. If you are someone who wants to be more private, this can be tough.

Chemotherapy and some forms of radiation can cause hair loss. Total hair loss is not a given and there are some chemo cocktails that don't affect the hair as much as others. There are measures to reduce the amount of hair loss, but nothing is a guarantee. We don't just lose the hair on our heads. I mourned the loss of my eyebrows and lashes more than what was on my head but not so much the other places that turned out as smooth as a baby's butt. No Brazilian bikini wax needed. I could cover my head but learning to draw on eyebrows wasn't easy for me. Plus, they never grew back as thick as they once were.

We lose 40 to 45 percent of our body heat through our heads and that needs attention. I, for one, was cold all the time and needed warmth but there are others who have more hormonal affects and felt like they were frying when wearing wigs. I was going through chemo in the winter which played a part for me, so the climate where you live matters. The bottom line is that many of us battle for ways to adapt to losing our hair.

Some approach hair loss proactively by having hair cutting parties or some kind of a ceremonial release of their hair. *It's more like a statement that my hair goes when and how I say so.* Cancer doesn't get to take this away from me, too. There are chemo cooling caps that some like to try to avoid losing hair at all. I can't speak to those because I never tried them.

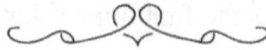

I was told to wait to cut my hair before starting chemo because some women don't lose it all and it may just thin a bit. My hair is baby fine and thin anyway, but I held off on cutting it. About two weeks after my first round of chemo, I was shedding hair worse than any dog could have. I woke each morning and carried my pillow outside to shake off the hair. I was still trying to cook meals, so we probably ate a good portion of it.

One day when my husband was at work, I got the bright idea to shave it off myself. One of my favorite power woman movies was GI Jane with Demi Moore as the first female Navy SEAL candidate. In one scene, she grew frustrated with her long hair, went into an empty barber shop and with a pair of hair clippers, sheared her head. It was a really sexy and powerful scene. I gathered up my stuff and did my own recreation of that movie scene. That's when I realized Demi Moore and I have nothing in common.

The first pass of fine hair drifted to the floor and my heart fell with it. I told myself it's just hair and it will grow back. My eyes raised to my reflection in the mirror, and I took in my sallow complexion and post-apocalyptic, nuclear fallout survivor hairdo and I started to cry. It wasn't just my hair. It was so much more. Yeah, I grew stronger and eventually I totally rocked head scarves, but in that moment, surrounded by locks of my hair about my feet, I grieved.

If Cancer is a Gift, Can I Return It?

"You don't look sick."

Remarking on someone's appearance with anything but a well-worded compliment is dangerous territory at best. It is better to say something positive instead of bringing attention to the negative. For instance, don't say something like "You don't look like crap" if a simple, "You look good" will work. Backhanded compliments like this example feel judgmental. The immediate reaction is to feel you have to justify what you need because of cancer. The effects of your cancer may not be visible to others but that doesn't invalidate how you feel or what allowances you need to make for yourself. We don't have to prove we have cancer by looking or acting a certain way. If someone wants to doubt your cancer experience, they can, but not to your face.

If you don't personally have cancer, please don't offer suggestions or advice. Despite all the best intentions, no one wants, needs, or appreciates unsolicited advice under any circumstances and especially not at a time like this. If you are the one who is bursting at the seams to inform a BC veteran about what or how they should do, feel, or think in any way about their experience and you can't stop yourself, ask if they want to hear your suggestion. Don't get your feelings bent out of shape if they don't. If you get the okay to spill your beans but their eyes are sending the I-wish-you-wouldn't message, please back off, change the subject, and keep your ideas to yourself. They are probably thinking that once you have actually gone through cancer and have advice to give, they will be more likely to appreciate it.

If you are the recipient of unwanted advice, this is where Teflon skin is great to develop. I got this idea from a BC veteran and friend who talked about how this is a time in your life that you just need drama, passive aggressive remarks, insults, and yes, unwanted advice to slide off without leaving a mark. Getting upset or angry with the person draws too much energy that you don't have to spare. Maybe the person is well-intentioned but ignorant as to what to say or not say, or even if the person is president of the Association of Spiteful Sociopaths (ASS), you do not have to take it personally. You also do not have to educate them, try to get them to see your side of the story, or explain anything at all.

I learned a lovely response to unwanted advice from an elderly lady that I, as her nurse, was trying to give her. I was advising her how to stay safer in her home. She and I both knew fully well that she had no intention in taking my advice, but she was too nice to say so. She just wanted me to shut up, so she said, "Thank you for that." End of conversation.

"My friend's mother had breast cancer... but she died."

There is a phenomenon where people, in a misguided attempt to connect with you, feel compelled to tell you horror stories. If they haven't had cancer or don't know better, they will blurt out anything they have read or heard about cancer or list those they know who have had it. The trouble is that they include almost exclusively the ones who didn't make it. How on Earth anyone can think it is a good idea to tell horror stories to someone facing a challenge is beyond me, but there it is.

If you want to show caring and connection to someone going through a difficult situation, listening is the best option. The greeting of "Hi, how are you?" has been so overused that everyone knows the person asking neither expects nor *wants* a real answer. Most people ask and keep on walking past. Actually asking and waiting for the answer is one of the easiest ways to truly connect and show your compassion. Make eye contact. You might get a fine-thank-you-for-asking answer, but they will feel seen and know you care.

It is so easy to feel invisible when you get a cancer diagnosis. People flock to you at first with condolences and vague offers of help that never materialize. Then, as you start to show signs of any treatment, the opposite happens. Some people start to acknowledge the reality of cancer in their lives because if it can happen to you, it can happen to them. They will struggle to be around you because of their own fears about cancer. These people make excuses to not get together with you, stop answering your messages, or not "like" your Facebook posts. Even though it is hard to *not* take this personally, we are not responsible for how others choose to act.

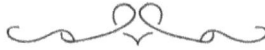

When I was first diagnosed with breast cancer, I was hungry for some sign that I could come out of this okay. Several times in the early days, I had coworkers and acquaintances come up to me out of the blue and start telling me about a cousin's friend who had a neighbor with an aunt who got breast cancer. I would hear them out and ask if everything came out okay. Every single time, and I mean Every. Single. Time. they would look a bit abashed and tell me no, the person died. How is it humanly possible that they would think I needed to hear that?

The last time this happened to me, a coworker walked up to me and started in with that familiar intro of "My hairdresser's mother…"

I held up my hand and said, "If this story doesn't have a happy ending, I don't want to hear it." It must not have because she stumbled over her words, grew silent, and then turned around and walked off.

I felt like I took a bit of my power back that day.

"You have to stay positive."

No, you don't HAVE to stay positive. You have to do a lot of things because of having cancer but staying positive isn't one of them. Yes, it is a good goal to strive for but keep in mind you have the choice to be present to whatever you feel in the moment.

No one stays positive all the time. If they say they are, maybe drugs are involved or a level of enlightenment I've not experienced yet. Real people have real feelings, and it is okay to feel your real feelings no matter the consequences. True, you might need to temper the expression of your feelings to not get fired or commit homicide but stuffing down their emotions is what leads many people to get in those situations in the first place. If the reality of cancer has done anything for me, it is to show me how my social mask was hiding far too much in the effort to be accepted.

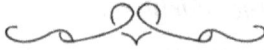

Sometimes people sent me cards that had words of encouragement and I loved them. Then there were times that people sang out perky "Keep your chin up" messages and I wanted to cry. I was so tired of being strong and I just wanted someone to be willing to be with me where I was, not keep telling me to feel something I couldn't. I wanted off the cancer roller coaster so badly, but that wasn't happening. I wanted to tell them they could trade places with me for a while and see how "up" their chin could be.

"I haven't been working since my diagnosis and have really bad chemo brain. I swear some of my friends think I'm taking a career break or just chilling out at home."

Here is where the competition with other breast cancer veterans and with yourself comes in. If you have identified with your career or the level of work you get done, having that wiped out leaves you struggling to know who you are and what your purpose is. I was a nurse forever and being forced to retire early was devastating. If I wasn't a nurse anymore, who was I? I wrapped my identity far too tightly around the fact that I have worked in some capacity since I was sixteen. I was officially out of work but didn't have the energy or mobility to enjoy it. It is easy to think someone is judging you, when actually you are. Even if they are thinking you are at home on the couch binge eating popcorn, let them. This is your time to heal, however you need to do it. Being home on the couch watching daytime TV and eating whatever you can, just may be what you need.

Every story about someone who accomplished magnificent things while you stayed curled up in the bed waiting to feel better is another mark against the mental scorecard. We all want to breeze through this process and be that person but not many of us get to be. The key is to stop expecting ourselves to match what we think others do. And it's crucial to not beat ourselves up for being unable to do what others expect of us. If you are the marathon runner or are inspired by the feats of others, I salute you. I was pleased to make it to the bathroom in time.

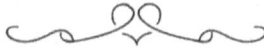

My nursing supervisor had breast cancer a few years before me. She regaled me with stories of how she worked and took mini breaks lying on the exam tables whenever she could. It was a lot of encouragement for me until I turned out to be one of those who couldn't work during chemo. She had told me that she worked the entire time and I made that to mean I was supposed to also. Only my brain had turned to mush. I couldn't get the energy to fight my way out of the fog that took up residence in my brain. My job was pretty easy in all honesty. My responsibilities were manageable, but I lost the ability to do my job with compassion. I was so drained; I couldn't even feel.

Then my white blood cell count dropped out. That morning, I dragged myself out of bed nearly in tears wishing I could have just a few more minutes before being forced to get up. Everything hurt, even the eyebrows that fell out long ago. Not realizing what was different in my body, I decided to call in sick, again. I could hear the disappointment in my supervisor's voice. She was going to have to either cover for me or cancel all my appointments that day. She asked me if I was sure I had to call in and guilt tore a hole in my conscience. Making it to work regardless of how I felt was one of the bragging points of my entire working career. I hesitated a bit until a wave of bone crushing pain seized me. I told her I was sure.

I got my husband to take me to the ER where I got an IV and some meds that took my pain away. There was a shaky young student nurse who was assigned to put my IV in and I was okay with that. My veins are huge and I'm a good confidence builder for learning students. The student nurse put the last piece of tape down and finally took a breath. That's when I told her she did a really good job and that I'm a nurse practitioner. She nearly fainted.

After my blood work came back and the pain was gone, I felt great! I could easily go to work. Or maybe that was the morphine talking. The IV came out and the resident physician shooed me out the door. Then, in passing, she said that my white blood cell count was rock bottom and that was probably why I hurt so badly all over. Who knew? Not me, even though I probably should have. Chemo had me in such a fog, I couldn't even figure out what was going on inside of me, much less what was going on with my patients.

It was a good thing I didn't go to work; my white count was dangerously low which would have left me vulnerable to all the colds and "bugs" that my clients seemed to always have. My nursing supervisor was still unimpressed.

———————

Suggestions like "You should learn another language" or "Try this advanced Excel course online" just don't help. Some days I can barely tie my shoes.

"You can't use chemo brain as an excuse forever."

The American Cancer Society refers to chemo brain as the mental cloudiness or lack of mental clarity that people can experience before, during, or after cancer treatment. It is described as having trouble finishing tasks, concentrating or focusing attention, or learning new skills. It can interfere with the ability to perform usual activities like school, work, or social activities. At best, these activities seem to take so much more mental effort than before.

Even though it is sometimes mistaken for dementia, chemo brain is not the same. In some cases of dementia, mental exercises help with memory, reasoning, and the speed of processing information. In my experience taking care of many people in treatment, when a someone's energy gets low or they are really stressed, forgetfulness and the feeling of just not being able to think straight happens. What is needed is a return to the best health status possible. Rest, sleep, stress reduction, and good nutrition all play a huge part in management. Demands to perform as before or judgment from others or yourself makes it more difficult. Chemo brain isn't a permanent situation unless there are additional underlying problems that need medical attention. It just feels permanent.

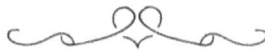

A few years after my chemo was in the rearview mirror, I was again on Dr. Makhoul's table for a follow-up exam. I complained about still feeling spacey and forgetful and blamed it on chemo. He said that I couldn't anymore; it had been too long.

Because I hold this doctor in such high esteem, I just smiled and let it go. If I want to blame a cloudy day or my coffee getting cold on having had chemo, I most certainly will.

"At least you got a free boob job."

Reconstruction of breasts after mastectomies is not remotely similar to a free boob job. For one, it comes at an incredibly high price: your natural breasts. Reconstructed breasts, depending upon the specifics and location of the cancer within the breast, the type of reconstruction, implants, and skill of the surgeon vary so much it would be impossible to cover all the potential outcomes here.

Nerves and muscles are unavoidably and permanently affected during surgeries causing them to be initially very painful and numb at the same time. Some women experience a deep itching sensation that can't be scratched. If you scratch your nails over the thin skin, you can potentially damage it. You can only feel pressure of your nails but not anything like an itch-relieving scratch. Nor can you feel any sexual or pleasurable sensations any longer. In fact, when my husband tried to fondle my reconstructed breasts, it was intolerably painful. At the very least, it was so uncomfortable that I would push him away causing him to feel rejected. He soon stopped trying which didn't do our relationship any favors. Sex for us had to become making the best of what I had left while avoiding any contact with my breasts. The normal physical sensations of the breasts never return. Just like phantom limb syndrome, there is a memory of how your breasts once felt, but it is faint.

I could never get past how cold and dead my reconstructed breasts felt. They looked dead, also. The skin over my left implant was purple and mottled, with incredibly poor blood supply and my nipple was a weird shade of gray. I couldn't stand to look at it. I turned away from any mirror to avoid seeing my body when undressed. My husband always tried to make me feel good about my body and never did I see him react negatively to the sight of my breasts, but my heart shattered every time anyway.

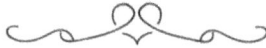

⌒⌒⌒

The first bath after getting my implant was a real shock. I got undressed and sank back into the warm, comforting water. I risked a glance down at my breast only to see that it looked deflated like a collapsed tent. I shot upright and my boob popped out. I laid back and it collapsed again. The thought that ran through my head at that point was that my husband was not going to get to see my breast... ever again.

Of course, that wasn't how life played out but I never got past that revulsion of how my breast looked in general but more so when I laid down. This wasn't even remotely close to what I expected. I hoped for the best, feared the worst, and expected something in the middle. This far exceeded the worst of my fears. This was my "free boob job."

Another problem with this free boob job is that rarely does one surgery reach the best results. Sometimes it takes a series of surgeries with all the potential problems such as infection, pain, and recovery time required to get the best aesthetic outcome.

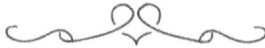

⌒⌒⌒

After a mammogram of my remaining breast a year after my initial mastectomy, I got news of a suspicious lump in my remaining breast. I had to go through another round of biopsies and agonizing waiting to see what it turned out to be. This time was worse because I knew what I was in for if I had to start treatment again. I had just finished my course of Herceptin infusions, every three weeks for a year. While they weren't as bad alone as when they were in a combined chemo drug regime I took for the first six months, I always felt gray and listless. The chance that I was going to have to go through this whole nightmare again was terrifying.

It turned out that the new lump was benign, but I was done. I asked for my remaining breast to be removed. I had a convoluted hope that if I had the failed implant replaced and got an implant on the right to match, I might have symmetry and nicer-looking breasts. Again, I failed to fear the worst.

The skin of my left breast was even a darker purple than before and had what looked like gouges streaking across it. Maybe a bear got in the operating room and took a swipe at me. The right was a normal color and permanently erect nipple which is about all I can say good about it. Without breast tissue, there has to be some acellular donor tissue placed between the implant and the skin for padding. Padding was placed around the sides of the breast mound but not under my retained nipple so I had a large, triangular crater in the middle. No way could this be described as normal. The shape of that crater and my single erect nipple was visible through my clothes and while I could hide it with a bra, they were too painful to wear.

My experience with breast implants was not good which is the understatement of the year. I've met other women, even with the same plastic surgeon as I had, who said they were happy with their outcomes. My experience is only my experience and not a judgment about whether or not to have reconstruction. I personally feel I was not fully aware or informed correctly of the complications and side effects. There was no discussion of what to expect or *potential health hazards of breast implants and the multiple surgeries that may be required to achieve an acceptable outcome. I was told they were completely safe.*

There was a general push to get reconstruction, as if that would repair my feminine body image. It felt like I was to get reconstruction as a matter of course, why wouldn't I? Since I was still reeling from the shock of my diagnosis of cancer, I just robotically did what I was told. It never even occurred to me to consider going flat. I metaphorically climbed up and planted my butt on the medical system conveyor belt, giving all my power to Those Who Knew What Was Best For Me.

Over the following years, my health spiraled down. My shoulders froze up. I was in constant pain with the energy level of a sloth. I could no longer use a vacuum, hang clothes up in a closet, fold a sheet, or do my job, forcing me into early retirement. I had a litany of health problems I couldn't find answers to. My breast surgeon and plastic surgeon left their respective practices, and I dropped through the cracks of follow-up.

Finally, I began to suspect there was something wrong with my implants. I sought out a reputable plastic surgeon and met him with the intent to have my implants removed. I didn't want any reconstruction. I wanted to just go flat. I felt that I could wear protheses if I chose. Those implants never felt like my body and once I had the chance to get them out, I couldn't wait to get rid of them.

In the process of getting ready for surgery, my breast ultrasound and MRI showed a ruptured silicone implant. The level of deterioration of the ruptured implant convinced me that I had been soaking up toxic chemicals for a very long time. Soon after removal, I felt so much better and regained use of my arms and vitality again.

If anyone could say I got a free boob job, this was the one that I was grateful for. Yes, I sometimes (but rarely) miss my pre-cancerous breasts, but I'll never miss those damned implants.

Can You Believe People Actually Say These Things?

"You're triple negative? OMG! That's a death sentence!"

"Did they tell you how long you have to live?"

"You know, cancer is anger turned inward."

"What is your prognosis?"

"Cancer is basically like a cold these days."

"Breast cancer is not a real cancer."

"You are so lucky because it could have been so much worse."

"You have to die of something."

"Didn't you just lose your mom to breast cancer, too?"

"Breast cancer isn't the death sentence it once was."

My personal favorite:

"You have the devil in you to have cancer and are ignorant in the Lord to not have gotten perfect healing."

I'm trying to imagine in what universe it is okay to say some of these things but I'm coming up empty handed. With the exclusion of people who sincerely struggle with social skills and maybe young children, it is clearly wrong for someone to remark or ask about your cancer or prognosis. Apparently, that didn't stop several people, or I wouldn't have had these examples and more. However, the important thing is learning how to handle these types of hurtful and insensitive remarks.

First of all, it is important to have healthy boundaries around your physical, relationship, and spiritual limits. This means knowing what is or isn't okay for someone to say to you or ask of you without feeling the need to over-explain, blame, or become defensive. Many are conditioned to have poor or no boundaries, usually due to past trauma or events that challenge their perceptions of their own self-worth. This was certainly true in my case. A low sense of self-worth keeps people in a loop of taking whatever people dish at them in order to prove their value and be accepted. If this describes you, know that you are in good company, but you have what it takes to break free.

Maybe you are a person who associates boundaries with being mean. If you were raised by or around a person who took boundaries to an ugly level, it's very possible to feel that saying no is not safe. Later, when you need to develop your own boundaries, the desire to not do to others what you experienced will compel you to avoid setting boundaries at all. Trying to keep others around you happy, being afraid of making them angry or upset, feeling guilty or overly responsible for other people's feelings—all are boundary pitfalls.

If you need help setting boundaries, you can try some of these measures:

- ❖ **Start small.** Little wins build confidence and set the stage for people to know you have limits. Try saying no to some small request or politely decline to listen to someone's horror story about cancer. A statement to the effect that you choose to focus on the positive will stop most with minimal drama.

- ❖ **Trust your intuition and body instincts.** If something feels off, it is. Trying to rationalize people's actions or words weakens your boundaries. Acknowledge your internal signals as loving personal guidance for yourself.

❖ **Let go of what you believe people will think.** Usually when someone is called out for a mistake, no matter how kindly, they will react with remorse, embarrassment, or defensiveness. You are not responsible for how they react. The only thing you have control of is how you react to whatever they say or do.

❖ **React but don't be reactive.** What you feel is your business. You have every right to feel whatever you do when you hear misspoken words. The goal is to choose to respond in a healthy way, not be reactive. If we don't feel free to own our emotions, we instinctively push back or feel hurt, angry, defensive, or conflicted. Not allowing ourselves permission to own our emotions causes us to react. When we are reactive, we say, do, and feel things that only cause us more pain in the long run.

❖ **Stay firm and confident**. You don't have to apologize, explain, or educate the person unless you feel it is right to do so. If you find yourself oversharing or justifying what you feel, take a breath and tell yourself that you deserve your privacy.

❖ **Be clear in your own mind what you want and what your priorities are.** Knowing what you want to say yes to helps you to say no to what you don't want.

❖ **Develop boundaries.** In the effort to respond appropriately to inappropriate remarks or questions, it's important to establish and maintain healthy boundaries. Every time you overlook an insensitive remark, it builds up inside causing you to overreact to the next remark. When you finally blow, it gets ugly. It's typically not directed at the person who started this mess but at someone you feel safer to let it out upon. Then you end up apologizing for hurting them.

These are some things that helped me:

- ❖ **Try to see from their perspective.** Sometimes it helps to lessen the sting if you look at the intentions of the person. Remember that the remark still hurts, and it is okay to be upset.

- ❖ **Try humor if that is your style.** Some BC veterans report that simply staying positive for others helped them to stay positive themselves. My bionic boob story helped me out of sticky situations.

- ❖ **Ignore them.** Walking away sends a clear message. So does silence. If you have to continue to interact with the person or persons, you can change the subject. That lets them know you are not open to the present interaction.

- ❖ **Stand up for yourself and make your needs known when you feel like it.** Telling someone a remark was hurtful or inaccurate sometimes is necessary. You have the right to your feelings. Be honest and authentic in your response. I-statement communications are helpful. (For example, I feel _____ when you say/ask/do _____.) You state your feelings while acknowledging, not attacking, their words or actions. Again, they may respond with defensiveness or passive aggression but that is their problem, not yours. You do not have to defend your feelings, just state them.

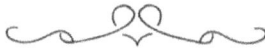

While waiting for my first surgery, I had several people come up to me with various degrees of mournful expressions to tell me how awful they felt that I was going to have a mastectomy. While it was nice that they cared enough to talk to me about it, I was tired of the long faces reminding me to be worried.

One day at work, there was a break between patients, and I walked out into the hallway to move around a bit. A nurse came up to me with a sad expression and said how awful it was that I was going through this and having a mastectomy. I responded that it would be, but I am getting a bionic boob. She started smiling and asked me what kind of weapon I was getting. Laughing, I told her to not piss me off because she didn't want to find out. Being rescued by a bit of humor was tons easier than constantly dealing with the gravity of my situation.

"You are so strong; I couldn't do it."

"I understand. I once had a bad mammogram."

Another human phenomenon is the need to make things about themselves. I'm not talking about pure narcissism, which is excessive self-absorption to the exclusion of all else. I'm referring to how people relate to external events by configuring them into how *they* would feel or react if they were in the same situation. This is perfectly natural and generally no problem unless you are the one who is in the undesirable situation.

When you are needing support, you don't need to be thinking about how someone else would handle what you are going through. Also, there are times when you don't feel strong and someone remarking on how strong or resilient you are adds more pressure to be that way. It takes a huge amount of energy to stay strong, and sometimes, you need to feel okay to not be.

You will also find some people show up with a bit of unnatural or morbid interest in how you are doing. Even though they don't come out and say it directly, they seem to be watching you like some research project to see how you do. It feels like you're under a microscope and they are taking notes. In my experience, some people made remarks to me that implied they wanted me to reassure them I would be okay. Not for my sake, though, but to make them feel they could survive if they were in that situation. If I could do it, maybe they could too. This was a huge energy drain for me. I had barely enough energy to get through the day and having to be strong for them was too much. Soon, I learned to feel an energy drain coming toward me and I would practically turn and run the other way.

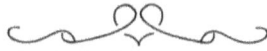

Working in different county health clinics brought a lot of personnel into my life. One nurse in particular would come up to me with a mournful look on her face and say something to the effect that she didn't know how I could do it, that she just didn't think she could handle what I'm going through.

Standing there with my professional mask cemented in place, I'm thinking, I can't either. I've changed my mind. I don't want cancer so I'm just not going to have it. I want a do over. Only I wake up every day and force myself out of bed into clothes, eat something, not because it tastes good but because that keeps me from passing out, and put one foot in front of the other until the second I can sit down. I don't have a choice.

She wouldn't have a choice either. She would buck up and force herself out of bed just like I did. She can do anything I can. She just doesn't want to be forced to do so. Can't say I blame her there, but giving up isn't an option, so you have to function whether you are strong or not. Quitting wouldn't change anything except how I get through the day. I still have bills and people depending upon me. I can dream about giving up all day, but I would still be struggling with the fact I have breast cancer. I'm not getting that do over.

"Well, that is all behind you now."

"It's in the past and time for you to move on."

Easy for someone else to say. Perhaps there are some people who have no fear of reoccurrence. Many of us fear that if cancer happens once, it can happen again. As much as you get caught up in life and forget about cancer, the possibility of reoccurrence sits in the darkness and waits for an opportunity to rear its ugly head.

This is when the exercises to stay in the moment help the most. We cannot control the future nor change the past, so staying present in the moment is the safest place to be. Being told to "move on" comes out more like "suck it up, buttercup" and serves no one. It is incredibly disrespectful of what the BC veteran has gone through.

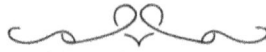

My first mammogram of my remaining breast came a year after my mastectomy and final Herceptin treatment. I had lost some weight and the mammogram appeared a bit changed from the previous one. I got called back for another biopsy of a suspicious area. Getting called back used to be a regular, routine occurrence to examine a benign area. That is until the last benign area turned out to be breast cancer. So all the fear the lizard brain could dredge up was choking me.

I went through all the tests and biopsies like a zombie while still trying to work. Just having to go through the whole process again was excruciating. The expected call with the results from the radiologist came while driving to work on the interstate. He had an incredibly upbeat tone of voice as he said he had good news. "The area was benign, so just come back in six months for another diagnostic mammogram."

I ended the call and thought, Another mammogram in six months. I don't think I can do this again.

Tears started falling down my cheeks and I was shaking violently. No, I can't go through this again. I can't have another mammogram. I won't do it. This was me having an emotional breakdown barreling down the highway at seventy-five miles an hour. This call was my supposed good news.

"For me, the hardest part was friends not saying anything or not coming around for support. Cancer isn't contagious, people!"

"Let me know if there is anything I can do to help." Then they would disappear.

When an initial catastrophe happens, general compassion and caring are brought out in most people. The ones closest to you may become your cheering squad while others disappear in a cloud of smoke. This is a time when true friends show up in your life and the fair-weather friends disappear.

This happens among family members, too. As hurtful as it is, this is a time to be glad to be rid of the shallow relationships and grateful for the ones who stick by you. We have probably all lived some parts of our lives creating shallow relationships. That's okay because we can choose different for ourselves going forth. However, if people disappear on you, it is about them, not you. Some will be afraid of the presence of cancer and others are tied up in the work of their own lives and can't give you what you need.

There comes a time when the support from other dwindles and you can feel lost or abandoned. The effects of cancer and treatment last a lot longer than the ability for others to provide you a support system. They get caught up in the drama and work of their own lives and simply do not have energy to spare for you.

This doesn't mean you do not matter. Nor does it mean it is wrong to continue to need support. It just means the support you need may have to come from a different direction.

Vague offers for help that never materialize can and will happen. Most even have honest intentions to help in some way but when it really comes down to it, they fold. Not following through on an offer to help will make them feel guilty so they will probably run at the sight of you. Again, this is not personal. Social etiquette is ingrained in many, so they are compelled to offer help even if they hope it is not needed of them.

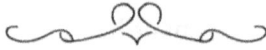

⁙

One of the more difficult things to ask a BC veteran, "Is there anything I can do for you?"

I was too tired to think of anything most of the time, so I generally gave a no, but thanks anyway response. It was really tough when someone asked, and I had something for them that they weren't counting on me needing. The surprised looks flashed across their faces and then an equivalent of, "Oh, gee golly, would you look at the time! I gotta go do this thing..."

If you have a real desire to help out in some way but are clueless as to how, try the statement, "I want to help, and this is what I can do..." A statement like this offers what is within your limits and lets the one going through this know you are there for them and can help in a specific way. It also takes the decision away from the person with the chemo-addled brain and lets them know you are there to help.

I didn't have little ones and was fortunate enough to be able to rest without eyeballs looking at me wanting something all the time. Well, except Maggie, who watched me like a hawk for the nanosecond I could move and then was casting doggie-ESP brainwaves at me to take her for a walk. For BC veterans who still have to function as moms and coworkers, just knowing that someone might be willing to pick up kids after school or come get them for a playdate must be huge.

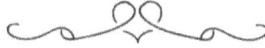

It was during my toughest chemo days that someone selflessly helped me in ways I didn't know I needed. Cathy, a neighbor who I knew in passing, became one of my biggest supporters and friends. She drove past my house on her way to and from work, so she started dropping off tokens that I truly appreciated. A plate of cookies I couldn't eat but my husband could enjoy would end up on my doorstep. Or she'd leave a small basket of magazines and a cozy throw or new gown. All of these would magically appear on my doorstep followed by a text to look out my door after she left. She intuitively knew I didn't have the energy to socialize and making conversation was too much work at the time.

I really didn't know her that well, but this was definitely a person I wanted to get to know. Today, I am honored to be able to say I can call her my bestie.

So, What *Can* You Say?

I got asked by a concerned coworker of a person just starting chemo about what to say to someone who is going through a cancer diagnosis and treatment.

My first response was "as little as possible." Then, I thought I best clarify that somewhat. Going through chemo for me was variable. Right after a treatment, I was not up for visits, writing email, conversation, responding to texts, or any human interaction for that matter. The days fluctuated from tough to dear-God-when-is-this-going-to-end tough. People stayed away in general during those days and that was good. Making nice was just too hard. I was glad my husband worked, and I didn't have to talk to anyone other than Maggie. As time passed after my last chemo treatment, I had days when I missed having someone to talk to— not bad enough to actually leave the house and seek people out, but I mildly wished Maggie was capable of more than one-sided conversations.

I think it's a good idea to let the one in treatment decide if, when, and where. Let them know that is what you are doing, too. Informing is always good.

"I'm open to visiting you when you feel up to it, but I'll wait to come over until you tell me."

Texting is great but only in statements that do not require a response.

"I'm thinking of you."

"Sending prayers."

"So sorry you are going through this."

"Sending love and light." But only if you mean it.

Avoid texting questions like "How are you?" whenever possible because it forces the person to actually have to think about how they are and decide if they should respond honestly or not. Sometimes, I didn't have the energy to text back.

If you are able to help, please do so, but offer specifics of what you are willing to do. Offers to pick up kids from school, getting something from the store because you are going anyway, laundry, or a simple casserole are great things. You don't have to worry about how it tastes.

When someone goes through chemo, everything tastes terrible but not having to fix food for the rest of the family is huge. Don't get hurt if the food offering isn't tolerated. Chemo does weird things to taste buds and that weird thing is different for everyone. A friend survived on Snickers bars, and while I dearly adore chocolate, during chemo it was the vilest substance I put in my mouth.

What I liked most was getting cards. They didn't have to be expensive, witty, or even with profound messages of hope and inspiration. I just felt the gift of being remembered. The cards really helped me get through the toughest of times. I still have them. I don't normally keep sentimental stuff like that, and never kept the wads of hair that came out of my hairbrush, but I kept those cards. They meant I wasn't forgotten.

Please do not underestimate the value of the smallest gesture. It may be someone's lifeline.

It's probably not a stretch to say that everyone wants to believe their life is of value to someone. We all want to matter, and to know that our lives have meaning beyond breathing air and taking up space. I desperately needed to know that no matter what happened to me, someone cared. I didn't want to be just an ant on the sidewalk that got stepped on.

Marching On

I have a dream...

Martin Luther King, Jr.

Between the lines on all the pages of this book is the message that you matter. This world is blessed that you were born and how you choose to live out your life is no reflection of your right to be here. Your value isn't about what you do or what happens to you but who you are at heart. Nothing that happens to you can change that. Getting diagnosed with breast cancer is not a measure of your worth nor punishment for the mistakes you've made. It is a massive life challenge that creates change. With any changes, there is loss and it is not only okay, but necessary to honor the grief you feel because of those losses.

When breast cancer happens, you are thrust into a chaos of emotions and fears. The ability to think rationally and objectively is rendered impossible until the threat is neutralized. To expect anything different of yourself or anyone going through this is ridiculous. It is tragic that people are expected—even forced—to make life-altering decisions at a time when logical thought processes are not possible. That sets people up for ill-advised decisions, regret, and disappointments down the road. You just have to do the best you can with what you have to choose from and know that no matter how it turns out, you gave it your best shot.

The mere act of receiving a cancer diagnosis is a traumatic event in itself. All attention immediately turns to physical survival, leaving the emotional and mental devastation behind to be dealt with later *if* it comes to be a problem. This line of thought is a catastrophic oversight. Your mental and emotional health are as vitally important as your physical health. My experience in the medical field has taught me that a person's healing is irrevocably linked to their mental and emotional health. You shouldn't have to fall apart before getting the help you need.

Speaking of help, we need to change our perception of what it means to ask for or need help. Asking for help is not a sign of weakness but rather a sign of great strength. It takes courage to ask for help because it takes courage to admit you need it. You also have to believe you deserve or are worthy of help to be able to receive it when it is offered. It's crazy to realize how hard it can be to ask for help. And when you are dealing with breast cancer, you shouldn't have to ask.

Change due to loss isn't always a bad thing. Even when something disastrous like breast cancer happens, you have the power to adapt and create a new perspective. Accepting yourself and your process and allowing yourself to receive support and guidance through the grief cycles can make this possible. Some changes need to happen. Toxic relationships need to be kicked to the curb and priorities need to be reevaluated. Change only gets scary when it shoves us out of our comfort zones. Keeping the known devil is tempting when facing the unknown.

Change needs to happen in the perception of the breast cancer experience, especially within the medical community. Focusing on physical treatment and recovery causes a tunnel vision that doesn't serve our best interests or higher good. You have a voice, should you choose to use it. Asking for attention and help for your mental and emotional needs in conjunction with or following your cancer treatment brings awareness to this oversight and helps make it easier for the person soon to be diagnosed. You can make a difference in the life of someone else. One voice can make that difference but the voices of the millions of BC veterans living with or recovered from breast cancer can start a revolution. Together we can create a glorious change.

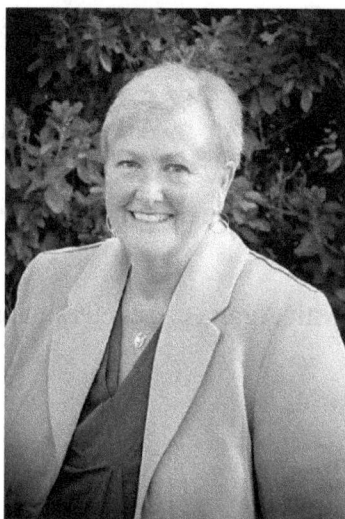

About the Author

After over 25 years in critical care nursing, her years in home health/hospice nursing in remote areas of the Ozark mountains of Arkansas, going back to school for her APRN, and working until retirement after a total of 40 years in nursing, Agalia Baker is no stranger to guiding people through their trauma and grief. However, none of her knowledge and experience softened the blow of being diagnosed with breast cancer herself.

Because of her experiences as a nurse and patient, she developed a passion to help others understand the emotional chaos that ensues after diagnosis. She hopes to shift the perception of the grieving process from a punitive viewpoint to an inspiring, healing path-way to processing trauma. She is also on a mission to bring attention to the emotional and mental health needs of every person diagnosed with breast cancer in order to initiate change in medical protocols. Being diagnosed alone is a trauma and everyone should receive the maximum support required in conjunction with any treatment regimes. Her personal and professional experience taught her that state of mind, mental outlook, and emotional strength improves patient health outcomes, quality of life, and survivorship.

She lives in a small town in Arkansas with the loves of her life: her husband of over 40 years, her two Standard poodles named Barney and Bailey, and Tuxi, the stray cat that came to dinner and stayed.

Stay connected with Agalia at bcveteran.com.

For more great books from Peak Press
Visit Books.GracePointPublishing.com

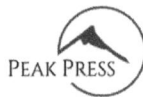

PEAK PRESS

If you enjoyed reading *If Cancer is a Gift, Can I Return It?* and purchased it through an online retailer, please return to the site and write a review to help others find the book.

www.ingramcontent.com/pod-product-compliance
Lightning Source LLC
Chambersburg PA
CBHW070331090426

42733CB00012B/2442